Under the Collar:
Simply Speaking
Audiobook Companion

A Adewusi, MD

L Hernandez, MD

OM MD

Opining Minions

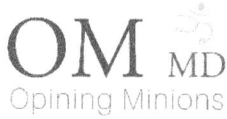

First Edition Copyright © 2020
Publisher: OMMD, Inc.

ISBN-13: 978-0-578-84723-8
Printed in United States

The conversations, events and locales in this work are derived solely from the author's recollections. To honor every individual's anonymity, including the author, the names as well as identifying characteristics of all persons and places have been changed. In all instances, the distillate of the conversations and events is accurate.

Cover Art and Design: OMMD, Inc.

THE POINT:

The common denominator among all difficult occupations is humans.

In every interaction, we humans bring our special brew of experiences, insecurities, strengths and weaknesses. Some compartmentalize (stow away) their insecurities while transforming their weaknesses into opportunities for new-found strengths. Some can project their anxieties onto others, creating a throbbing network of crippling fear and hostility. In such a network, each workday looms as a threat. In response to that threat, humans prepare to defend their time, their money, their self-perceptions through selfishness, passive aggression and hostility. Other humans act somewhere in between. On their best day, the other humans may be able to shelve their anxieties and proceed cooperatively, productively. On their exhausted days, they may spew bitterness from their lips or keypads.

Medicine, the supposed selfless occupation, has the greatest number of all three human styles with the greatest consequences when all three collide.

Effective patient care requires responsible colleague care.

This is not about polite exchanges and identifying implicit bias. This is not a tool to teach human decency. Human decency cannot be taught. A person either knows how to treat another person humanely or does not know. One is instinctively either humane or inhumane.

This conversation is about honing one's perspective of and respect for every player on the team so that the goal can be achieved – useful healthcare.

■ ■ ■

Simply Speaking is an audiobook abridgement to the analytical memoir *Under the Collar: Frank Conversations about Healing that Harms.*

"Hell is – other people! … Well, well, let's get on with it. …"
Huis Clos, Jean Paul Sartre

THE CONVERSATIONS

HOSPITALIST TO EMERGENCY PHYSICIAN

HOSPITALIST TO NURSE

HOSPITALIST TO ADMINISTRATION

THE END

A Clarification

Before delving into the conversations, several instances involve hospice care. Hospice practices have confused even practitioners. Below is a clarification and quick reference when needed.

. . .

So, what is hospice?

Hospice is ideal for someone in which inevitable death will soon occur regardless of any medical interventions provided to the patient.

Whereas the care for a patient with a nonterminal condition can be aggressive, uncomfortable, and downright painful at times, the goal of hospice is to keep the body comfortable until the body inevitably yields to death.

Under hospice care, patients are educated that hospitalization should be avoided, as hospitalization usually requires those aggressive treatments no longer beneficial to a dying patient. Even seemingly innocuous treatments with antibiotics can unnecessarily distress the body. (An example is an antibiotic's potential sequela Clostridium difficile infectious diarrhea that can erupt into toxic megacolon.)

The rare occasion in which hospitalization can be helpful for the hospice patient is one that relieves severe discomfort. For instance, a dying patient that newly develops severe abdominal pain caused by fluid retention may be temporarily admitted for removal of that fluid then discharged back to hospice care as soon as possible. The keynote here is: relieve discomfort, not resolve the illness.

Rather than seek emergency services during an episode of acute distress, hospice patients and families are advised to contact hospice first, *always*. Hospice can coordinate management of the acutely distressing condition which will circumvent unnecessary, uncomfortable hospitalization.

HOSPITALIST TO HOSPITALIST

getting through the night part I: What the Doc?!

> Amid the rampant opioid epidemic, protocols have been developed to minimize or avoid potentially harmful drug interactions. For instance, the combination of narcotics with benzodiazepines such as lorazepam (Ativan), diazepam (Valium), or alprazolam (Xanax) can lead to sudden death. Opioids are frequently coupled with antihistamines such as diphenhydramine (Benadryl) to lessen itching, a common side effect of narcotics. Antihistamines are equally effective whether administered orally or intravenously. Intravenously delivered antihistamines, however, not only relieve itching but also enhance opioid euphoria, intensifying addiction.

Mr. Mann was admitted for a "flareup" of his chronic medical condition that required treatment with IV narcotics. Mr. Mann refused to take oral diphenhydramine but finally relented to accept it orally after a forty-five-minute debate with hospitalist Jackson. Jackson insisted that he follow hospital guidelines. Jackson made sure the nurse witnessed the discussion and shared the restriction for oral diphenhydramine with the charge nurse.

Irked, the following morning, Jackson learned that the on-call nocturnist Wembley had been asked by the night nurse to switch from the oral diphenhydramine to the IV form, per Mr. Mann's request.

The very moment Jackson broached this issue, Mr. Mann harped, "If this is hospital policy to use oral diphenhydramine, why did another doctor on *your* team agree to change me back to IV?? I feel like this is only happening whenever *you* are my doctor!"

Silently exasperated, Jackson listened to Mr. Mann's defense. That one, cursory telephone order left Jackson defenseless.

. . .

The long and short of it:

Jackson tried not to use hospital resources to get Mr. Mann high. He secured a witness (the bedside nurse) and informed the authorities (the charge nurse) to prevent injection of the drug. Mr. Mann waited for Jackson to leave. Mr. Mann successfully exhausted the nighttime team (the skeleton crew) to push IV drugs.

Why did Wembley succumb?

Wembley must survive. He was outnumbered – patients, nurses, ED docs, specialists taking call from home. Becoming the night's yes-man ensures an easier shift.

It was only one night of narcotic enabling. It was just one night of positively reinforcing hospital policy defiance. It was just that one night when, in seconds, Jackson's authority to keep a problematic narcotic abuser at bay was evermore invalidated. (However, in reality, it is never just one night in which the skeleton crew dismisses collective policy for personal peace.)

Never mind that and disregard the damaging aftermath of egocentric medicine. Focus on its boomerang effect instead: Pretend Wembley is the daytime hospitalist and Jackson is the cross-covering nocturnist. Would it matter to Wembley when Jackson destroys all the work and wangling Wembley accomplished during the day? Why would it? Surely Wembley would ratify his own art – the practice of ME-dicine.

ehr: transparency or self-preservation

EHR stands for electronic health record. It is propagandized as open communication among healthcare organizations, practitioners, and patients. This open communication has been coined *transparency.*

Scrutinize the documents below for contradictions.

Author	Provider Type	Date of Service
Sam, MD	Hospitalist Medicine	XXX 20, YYYY

HOSPITALIST **PROGRESS NOTE**
Sam, MD
Hospital Day #0
PCP: No PCP

ASSESMENT AND PLAN
20-year-old woman with von Willebrand disease presented with severe, menorrhagia unrelieved by outpatient management
Principal Problem:
Menometrorrhagia
--persistent menometrorrhagia due to von Willebrand disease, failed outpatient management
--vaginal bleeding improved after DDAVP x 2 doses, but patient now with hyponatremia
--*tighten fluid restriction (1000ml/day) and monitor for worsening hyponatremia from DDAVP*
--Hematology Dr. Redd B Cell following
--*follow up repeat vWD labs*
Active Problems:
Von Willebrand disease (HCC)
--see above

Acute hyponatremia
--*due to DDAVP -- with dizziness*
--*fluid restrict and monitor – recheck at 1800 to ensure it is not worsening*

Migraine headache
--caffeine-withdrawal headache – Tylenol or motrin prn and routine AM coffee

See Orders.
VTE prophylaxis/Anticoagulation: ambulate
Diet Regular

DISPOSITION: home
Anticipated day of discharge: X/21/YY or X/22/YY

Author	Provider Type	Date of Service
Jim, MD	Hospitalist Medicine	XXX 21, YYYY

HOSPITALIST **DISCHARGE SUMMARY**
Admit date: X/18/YY 4:06 PM
Discharge date: Thursday, XXX 21, YYYY
No PCP

REASON FOR ADMISSION:
Patient presents with:
Infusion: sent by md for ddavp
FINAL DIAGNOSES:
Principal Problem:
Menometrorrhagia
--persistent menometrorrhagia due to von Willebrand disease, failed outpatient management
--vaginal bleeding improved after DDAVP x 2 doses, but patient now with hyponatremia
--*tighten fluid restriction (1000ml/day) and monitor for worsening hyponatremia from DDAVP*
--Hematology Dr. Redd B Cell following
--*follow up repeat vWD labs*
Active Problems:
Von Willebrand disease (HCC)
--see above

Acute hyponatremia
--*due to DDAVP -- with dizziness*
--*fluid restrict and monitor – recheck at 1800 to ensure it is not worsening*

Migraine headache
--caffeine-withdrawal headache – Tylenol or motrin prn and routine AM coffee

See Orders.
VTE prophylaxis/Anticoagulation: ambulate
Diet Regular

• • •

Find anything? ... Really? How so, when copy-and-paste is a flawless operation?

Fortunately, the progress note does not contradict the discharge summary. Still, is the discharge summary meant to regurgitate verbatim the inpatient note? If so, then is sending someone home with active problems and pending orders an appropriate discharge?

Whether the patient was sent home with active problems or whether Dr. Jim simply copied and pasted an inpatient note onto a discharge summary, both actions welcome weighty legal ramifications for Jim, his employer and the hospital at large – particularly during this era of transparent medicine. Why, then, would Jim jeopardize his license?

Imagine that Jim started his shift in the morning with more than 16 people to see, all completely new to him. He must learn the reason for admission and the treatment course for every single person; field questions about individuals of whom he knows nothing; see everyone before hour-long (at best) bedside collaborative rounds with the entire team (nurses, case managers, pharmacists, therapists and administrators); discharge everyone stable to leave the hospital before noon; update family members arriving throughout the day; discuss barriers to discharge with the hospitalist site leader; and lastly, empty, hydrate and feed himself to remain fit to function.

Now imagine the night before when Jim stayed up late with little Jimmy until the child's diarrhea settled. Finally resting his head at two in the morning, Jim blinks awake to an alarm alerting him to groom himself and the kids in time to report for his shift at 7 a.m. An email reminds him about the staff meeting from noon to two. A text message from his spouse reminds him to finish in time to pick up his other son, the littlest Jimmy, from daycare no later than 5:45 p.m. *and* be dressed for dinner with the parents at six. Jim is also reminded to keep his phone on vibrate during dinner until after seven (till he is no longer required to answer nurses' calls). Considering Jim's hefty docket, his cutting corners is not so alarming. His lack of responsibility is.

Jim is expected to be a responsible manifold being. He is not just a doctor: He is a partner, a father, a son, a friend, a provider for his family and a man. As a partner, he has a responsibility to harmonize, strengthen and enrich his shared life with another. As a father, he has a responsibility to rear his progeny to be the best individuals they can be. As a son, he has a responsibility to honor those who have cared for him with their good intentions. As a friend, he has a responsibility to reciprocate companionship, confidences and encouragement. As a family provider, he has a responsibility to satisfy the base layers of Abraham Maslow's hierarchy of needs. As a man, he has a responsibility to himself to reach the apex of that very hierarchy.

Now, as a doctor, he has the responsibility to accept his time-clashing life choices; to appropriately prioritize them as the setting dictates; and to fully, honestly, exhaustingly commit his noblest efforts every time he *chooses* to slip into that white coat.

hospice – not your everyday admission ... or any day

Ms. Mann, an 84-year-old woman with advanced dementia receiving hospice care was taken to the emergency room after suffering multiple seizures at home. Alarmed, her family revoked hospice measures to allow treatment for the seizures. Ms. Mann's dementia had progressed to where she could no longer feed herself, walk, communicate, recognize her family or engage in any activities that had previously defined her desired quality of life.

As uncontrolled seizures can be uncomfortable, a neurologist determined the medical cocktail to alleviate consequent suffering. The family confirmed their intent to allow Ms. Mann to die at home and remain comfortable as long as permitted. She was discharged home with prescriptions for the new antiseizure medications. Prior to discharge, Ms. Mann's daughter, her primary caregiver, spoke with the hospice liaison to ensure the supply of all necessary complements for at-home palliation (such as pain medications, sedatives, respiratory mediators, supplemental oxygen, a hospital bed, etc.). Her daughter also received information about contacting the hospice agency first for any acute crises any time of the day.

The very next day, Ms. Mann was brought back to the hospital emergency room for uncontrolled seizures. Her daughter had not yet picked up any of the antiseizure medications from the pharmacy. When she realized the seizures were recurring, she did not bother with the pharmacy and instead brought her mother back to the hospital. ER physician Herman treated Ms. Mann with IV medications and contacted Hospitalist Leslie to admit Ms. Mann. After reviewing the chart, Leslie, noting the hospice goal, explained to Herman that the issue was collecting the antiseizure medication from the pharmacy and initiating the home regimen. Leslie recommended advising the family to promptly pick up then start the medications at home. When asked her wishes for her mother, Ms. Mann's daughter expressed that she wanted her mother to remain at home with hospice care but would revoke hospice so that her mom could be hospitalized for seizure treatment. Concerned that Ms. Mann's daughter may benefit from further education about the services the hospice agency could provide, Leslie contacted their hospice liaison himself to request yet another discussion with the daughter. The hospice liaison offered 24-hour in-home care by hospice staff. The daughter agreed. The hospice liaison also arranged ambulance transportation to ensure Ms. Mann's safe return home later that evening.

Ms. Mann lay drowsily in the ER while awaiting her return home. She, like others after seizure episodes, was experiencing a prolonged state of drowsiness, called the postictal state. This postictal state can last for longer periods if multiple seizures occur in succession, as in Ms. Mann's situation. While she rested comfortably awaiting the ambulance transport, ER physician Herman now expressed concern that Ms. Mann would be too drowsy to take her antiseizure medications by mouth and insisted she be hospitalized for IV antiseizure medications. By this hour, after meticulously documenting the events, wishes and decisions, hospitalist Leslie had now left for the day. Hospitalist Boris accepted Herman's request. Boris started Ms. Mann on IV antiseizure medications, IV fluids for dehydration and other IV medications to control a fast heart rate. He attached her to a continuous heart monitor for the fast heart rate, consulted a cardiologist for the fast heart rate, and finally, consulted a neurologist for uncontrollable seizures.

The next day, hospitalist Irvin assumed care. The neurologist repeated that the previously prescribed antiseizure medications were most fitting. The cardiologist, who had idly followed Boris' lead, endorsed the cardiac monitor and IV medications until Irvin confirmed Ms. Mann's daughter's intention for hospice.

After two days of more meetings and deliberations among the doctors and hospice providers, it was decided that Ms. Mann would return home yet again. This time, she would have a specialized catheter through which medications could be administered rectally. Her discharge medications remained the same. Her daughter promised to pick up the medications from the pharmacy.

. . .

Good thing Ms. Mann was able to hold on for those four days in such an unfamiliar, unappealing, undesirable hospital room where strangers poke, prod and roll one this way then that way. Oh, digression!

– On to the practitioners:

Even when the ER physician loses sight of the goal, the hospitalist must stay the course to navigate patient and family through fear and confusion during unpredictable end-of-life passages. Boris needed to be the guide for the family and the example for Herman. Unlike Boris, Leslie attempted to prevent cyclic confusion among Ms. Mann's family members by emphasizing the importance of starting the antiseizure regimen immediately *at home*. Rather than spend hours educating, reaffirming and reconnecting hospice with the family, Leslie could have easily outfitted Ms. Mann in some hospital box within an hour or less. Discerning the true desires or intentions of people and reaching a clear, mutual understanding takes time – gobs of time. Boris probably knew that.

So, he cut to the chase: Boris set the patient up on *invasive* – pardon – *intravenous* fluids; he saw a heart rate and pushed *invasive* – pardon – *intravenous* rate-controlling medications; he tethered her to a machine and introduced her to another stranger, a cardiologist; he reintroduced her to a familiar unfamiliar, the neurologist. Then, he got her off his list, finished his shift and went home. Meanwhile, Ms. Mann served four days in the hospital.

Irvin comes along and attempts to restore Ms. Mann and family to their home. What a hero! Wait, what hero thinks comfort comes best rectally? Is rectal invasion not invasive? Well, when compared to metal penetration (a needle stick), a soft, malleable rectal catheter is favorable. Also, if smooth rectal suppositories are sanctioned to relieve abdominal discomfort from constipated and bloated bowels, a smooth rectal catheter that will deliver *anti-suffering* – pardon – *antiseizure* medications to someone who desperately needs them but cannot swallow them could be seen, like suppositories, as a noninvasive measure promoting comfort. Perhaps Irvin *is* a hero. Or, perhaps, Irvin is just a human being willing to put in the time to do the humane thing.

just in case medicine

Hospitalist Harold worked furiously on Mr. Mann's admission for seizure. Mr. Mann remained in a postictal state of confusion. The postictal (after seizure) state can last minutes to hours. Due to prolonged confusion, Mr. Mann required close monitoring. Harold clicked onto the seizure precautions option. These measures instruct staff to assess the patient frequently and ensure his safety should seizures recur. Included is a NPO order that restricts oral intake to prevent lung aspiration in someone not fully alert. Harold ordered IV fluids to preserve Mr. Mann's hydration.

Harold suddenly paused, gazed blankly in the air, then typed one final order:

"Consult the pulmonologist in case the patient aspirates."

■ ■ ■

What? ... *In case?* That is odd.

That must mean one should not leave one's home, *in case* he has a car accident. Another must not go to the park, *in case* he is struck by lightning. A third must never go to bed, *in case* he fails to wake. Or, maybe Mr. Mann must never eat again, *in case* he ever choked.

It might mean, one must refrain from practicing medicine, *in case* fear of sole accountability scares him.

veiled threats episode 2

Hospitalists Logistics:

Admitting versus Rounding Physician – At this facility, a patient is admitted by a dedicated admitting hospitalist. After admission day, the admitting hospitalist has no further involvement in the patient's care, and the patient is assigned to a rounding hospitalist. The rounding hospitalist treats the patient for the duration of his hospital stint then reassigns the patient to the next rounding hospitalist, and so forth, until discharged.

Test Orders – Whenever a physician orders a test, he is responsible for the results. If a patient is discharged prior to release of the results, the ordering physician either directly addresses them or arranges for the outpatient primary care physician to be notified about any outstanding test results.

It was the first of several days hospitalist Tate would serve as a rounding physician. As he worked, he returned a page from the laboratory department. Lab technician Brody reported highly abnormal lab results for recently discharged Ms. Mann. Now that Ms. Mann's results were final, Brody, noting that Tate had been her admitting hospitalist, decided to call him with the results. Tate recognized Ms. Mann as someone whom he had admitted last week. Tate explained that he had not been involved in Ms. Mann's care after admission, nor had he ordered the test. Tate scanned the electronic medical record and noticed that the rounding hospitalist who had both ordered the test and discharged Ms. Mann just happened to be today's admitting hospitalist. Tate directed Brody to contact the ordering physician.

Brody crisply replied, "Okay. I'll go ahead and record here that you refused to take information about your patient."

Annoyed, Tate answered, "A statement like that is implying that I chose not to do my job. I am kindly referring you to the doctor that can appropriately respond to your lab results. My name should not even be mentioned in your documentation. You need to call the actual provider and leave my name out of it!"

. . .

Well … Brody should.

It is understandable to pick the first name one sees, unburden oneself as quickly as possible and move onto the next task. Sure it is; but is that responsible? No.

With that in mind, should Tate have just relented, read about Ms. Mann's hospital course plus the reason for the test at discharge, and figure out how to proceed with the abnormal test result? No. Tate already had a newly adopted, full census for the day to read about and figure out how to proceed. In kind, Brody would likely have protested if someone attempted to burden him with his fellow technician's work. So why should Tate be scolded for not accepting someone else's responsibility when the responsible person is just a page away?

Still, Tate's response to Brody's passive aggression was callous. When insulted, it *is* quite tricky to be diplomatic and not defensive. Had Tate maintained an indifferent tone and skipped those last seven words, Tate would have been flawless in this exchange. Although a placid tone and conscientious wording would likely lead to the same end – both parties peeved with each other – there is merit in securing the upper hand.

busy is not new and no excuse

In his home, Mr. Mann suffered a cardiac arrest and was found unresponsive by his daughter. EMS promptly arrived to initiate resuscitation. The gentleman regained cardiac activity for only ten minutes before, once again, suffering a second arrest. In the emergency department, he required intubation as well as treatment for hypothermia. He never regained consciousness. Tests revealed that uncontrolled diabetes led to a severe hyperosmolar coma with blood sugar levels reaching an astronomical 5000 mg/dl (normal is 80-100 mg/dl); this coma led to the gentleman's cardiac and cognitive arrest.

Hospitalist Jake has never seen such blood sugar levels. (Even the endocrinologist had gasped!) Although massive doses of insulin are controlling Mr. Mann's blood sugar, his brain and kidney function still remain greatly compromised given the severe shock from both arrests. Jake scans this gentleman on life support with kidney failure and anoxic encephalopathy (brain injury due to low or absent oxygen flow). Scratching his head, Jake marvels that, unlike typical patients on life support, Mr. Mann does not require any sedation to tolerate the discomfort typical of mechanical ventilation. Also, ventilated patients gradually become more responsive within two to three days. Mr. Mann not only fails to wake by day four but has also begun *posturing* (tight extension and flexion movements indicative of severe brain injury). The neurologist notes nonexistent corneal (eye), cough and gag reflexes during his examination. Upon review of the EEG (electroencephalogram to test the brain's electrical activity), the neurologist determines Mr. Mann's condition is an "alpha coma" due to a prolonged state of oxygen deprivation in the brain, and, in fact, may already be "brain dead."

After numerous tearful discussions with Mr. Mann's loved ones, Jake prepares the family for the often confusing and unpredictable conclusion of physical life.

Following withdrawal of all life support and life sustaining measures, Mr. Mann will continue only those medications needed to keep his physical being comfortable. Jake clearly documents the family's request for comfort measures only.

Two days later, Mr. Mann exhibits small signs of responsiveness by moving his head when family says his name. He also faintly opens his mouth or weakly lifts a finger upon repeated commands. The hopeful family requests resuming life-sustaining treatments. Cross-covering hospitalist Ian answers the family's phone call. In an instant, without reviewing the medical record, Ian restarts IV fluids, seizure medications and antibiotics.

The next day, perplexed (and troubled by the emotional upheaval Mr. Mann's family will invariably endure due to the rash reversal), Jake plainly queries Ian.

> Jake: You started medications and full treatment on a patient on comfort care. This will not change his outcome.
>
> Ian: I did it because the family asked me to.
>
> Jake: Yeah, but did you review the chart to see what previous discussions and assessments had been made? Resuming treatment gives them the unrealistic expectation that he will get better and goes against the plan for comfort care. Which family member did you speak to?
>
> Ian: I don't know who it was.
>
> Jake: It took a long time for the family to make that decision for comfort care. One family member in particular was very unrealistic about the prognosis. Hopefully that wasn't the person you spoke to, but his wife, his legal decision-maker.
>
> Ian: Look, I get what you are saying, but it was a very busy night. I'm getting called in-between admissions and other cross-cover

calls. I did my best to appease the family and figured other concerns could be addressed in the daytime.

■ ■ ■

This incident illustrates several, grave tiers of harm. For simplicity, consider the impact the reversal of care can have on Mr. Mann and his family, then address the conflict between the two hospitalists.

Mr. Mann and Family

"Must we end his life?"

That is the interpretation of the customary question, "Will you withdraw life support today?"

Now, consider the series of discussions that preceded the decision to stop life support. The emotional toils prior to, during, and after Mr. Mann's transition from a life of independence to a ventilator-dependent existence then death can haunt all family members indefinitely. The burden weighs on not only the legal decision-maker but also on all individuals involved. Even mere witnesses will be affected by the entire ordeal. For those who feel as if they must choose to "kill" or "save" their loved one, any shred of hope that suggests life will instantly be adopted. No one wants the guilt of "giving up" on someone.

Therefore, providers must guide family and friends through contrary signs of hope and hopelessness. Providers cannot create or dictate life; but they can create realistic expectations to help others cope with the outcome should physical life expire. Realistic expectations begin with a thorough understanding of how an individual defines *quality of life* – and that takes time!

When faced with guilt, sometimes families need a remote, knowledgeable, sympathetic person to interpret what they are observing and, if fitting, to reassure them that they are not killing their loved one by withdrawing life support. They may need to be reminded about the kind of life their loved one once lived and would want to continue living.

(By the by, if someone's ultimate goal is to simply physically exist until life extinguishes, then providers must honor this person's definition. Providers must usher that individual and family into the next stages of long-term care to realize those wishes.)

The Hospitalists

Jake's and Ian's actions suggest different ideas about comfort care. Jake focuses on the prognosis. Ian focuses on symptoms. Jake's actions are patient centered. Ian's actions are family centered. Jake's approach was slow and cautious. Ian's approach was quick and decisive.

Now, before judging either's actions or approaches, note that Jake had an advantage by having numerous conversations over several days, while Ian had only one conversation for only one night. Considering Ian's disadvantage, there is no excuse for what appears to be a rushed act. Ian admitted during his confrontation with Jake that he had made a pressed decision. So, it is unlikely that, like the family, Ian too saw hope in Mr. Mann's responses. Also, Ian conducted his entire "assessment" over the phone and failed to examine Mr. Mann, which further lessens the likelihood the physician acted on hope. Rather, Ian's actions and confessions expose his desire to empty his pager no matter the detriment.

Floods of nurse and emergency room calls justify deferring nonemergent concerns, elective procedures or complicated matters to the daytime physician or team. Unfortunately, not all complicated matters can simply be hushed and tucked away until sunlight. There are a host of issues that will force a nighttime physician to juggle hospital admissions and nonemergent floor assessments. Had Ian taken the time to read the notes, lay eyes on Mr. Mann and address the family in person, he would have appropriately deferred that decision for Jake the next morning and would not have felt pressured to *appease* (translation: shut up) the family.

Appeasing patients and their families is not responsible medicine. Chasing patient satisfaction ratings while practicing substandard medicine is an insult to the Hippocratic oath. Compromising one's practice cheapens this oath, rendering it, in the end, a languid salutation.

the path of least inconvenience

Hospitalist Frank polishes his personalized electronic health record (EHR) templates. He routinely orders narcotic medications for every patient he admits to proactively address the most common complaint – pain. He tailored several electronic order presets to prevent interruptions from pages during his admitting shifts:

> For mild pain, patients receive a low dose of narcotics.
>
> For moderate pain, patients receive a higher dose.
>
> For severe pain, patients receive an even higher dose of narcotics.

With Frank's system, nurses can automatically drug anybody with slight discomforts. Nowhere in his template is an order for non-habit-forming pain relievers such as Tylenol or ibuprofen.

■ ■ ■

Efficiency is the dogma of all professions. Finding avenues to increase productivity while lessening obstacles to production (such as relentless pages) is a never-ending feat. Protocols and order presets have become a standard in electronic documentation to achieve maximum efficiency. Still, "checklist healthcare" has its limitations. There are several situations that must be consciously considered. Given the United States' rampant opioid crisis, assessing the appropriateness of narcotic treatments is one of those scenarios.

Explore how Frank's ease with unmonitored narcotic dosing furthers the opioid predicament: it encourages other providers to mechanically order narcotics with little regard for patients' long-term well-being. Soon, a culture of blind opioid pushing flourishes among providers. In no time, among the community of drug abusers, the hospital earns the distinction of a legalized crack house once those abusers learn that a little obnoxious nagging will guarantee their drug of choice. In essence, Frank unintentionally becomes a lawful drug dealer carrying a quiet pager.

Besides increasing the number of existing opioid abusers (and potential narcotic fatalities), Frank's practice, like an adroit dealer, recruits opioid-naïve individuals into the tragedy of addiction. If addiction does not occur, the risk for hospital-induced morbidity increases. Over-sedation, bowel immobility and respiratory depression are a few adverse conditions Frank can cause in opioid-naïve patients.

In both the opioid-naïve and opioid-versed populations, Frank's blanket pain management guarantees that mild discomforts or unusual complaints will be improperly treated. Protocol narcotic treatment of complaints can result in new problems, while masking the severity of the underlying problem. Frank's narcotic checklist misses opportunities to uncover the source of patients' ailments, improve or resolve their medical issue(s), and restore them to their everyday level of functioning.

Oh well ... at least his pager is not an inconvenience.

forget simon – what does the doctrine say?

Mr. and Mrs. Mann brought their eight-year-old daughter to the hospital for a fever that began two days after persistent nausea, vomiting and diarrhea. The concerned parents worried their daughter caught swine flu. Popularized by mass media as the next global demise, the notorious epidemic caused by the H1N1 influenza virus terrified many.

The little girl had severe dehydration, warranting hospitalization for supportive treatment with IV fluids until she could sustain oral intake of both food and fluids. Mr. and Mrs. Mann requested their child be tested for swine flu. Hospitalist Benson explained that her symptoms were classic features of a common viral gastroenteritis or the "stomach bug." The child had no muscle or joint aches, sore throat, congestion or cough that would suggest influenza or a similar illness. Benson also explained how the typical course and recovery from this common gastroenteritis can average one to seven days. Reassuringly, the hospitalist further added that their daughter would be closely monitored to ensure that she did not develop flu symptoms.

The following day, the girl's fever and vomiting subsided, but her nausea and diarrhea persisted, though with less severity. She tolerated fluids well but remained on IV fluids at a slower rate until the resolution of her diarrhea, which, Benson hoped, would occur by the next day. He updated the doting parents about their child's improvement and care plan.

Hours later, while preparing to evaluate a new patient, nurse Mark rushed to Benson's side warning, "Mr. and Mrs. Mann have been threatening to report you to the hospital administrator if you don't test their daughter for the swine flu!"

"But she doesn't have swine flu. She doesn't have influenza symptoms. And she's getting better with treatment for dehydration from gastroenteritis."

"Well," a dubious Mark emphasized, "I just thought I'd warn you."

Benson, a new residency graduate playing by the rules, again explained his reasoning to the parents and his certainty that the test would return negative for swine flu; but, to avoid trouble with the parents and administrative involvement, Benson ordered the panel for all testable influenza variants. As expected, the entire panel returned negative for any type of influenza.

The young girl's diarrhea resolved overnight. By morning, she tolerated solid foods without nausea, vomiting or diarrhea. Little Miss Mann was discharged home in excellent condition by lunch time.

. . .

It is rough for any newbie starting his career as a "rely-solely-on-your-own-judgement" attending physician. The inexperienced practitioner is bombarded with multitudes of uncertainties and fears. In addition to learning to trust the knowledge he has acquired from the latter half of residency, he must learn to follow his own lead (and only his lead if he is the sole physician for the service). The newbie must also figure out the common laws of each floor – those unwritten practices that are not industry standards but are performed, because "that's just the way it's done around here." With so many whirling unknowns and uncertainties, it is challenging for a new graduate to discern which requests or cautions are worth honoring. Benson illustrated this turmoil when he pitted his knowledge and instincts against aggressive parents and nervous nurse Mark. Simply clicking on a laboratory order to pacify the Mann family seems like a harmless act.

If months later, however, Mr. and Mrs. Mann reviewed the hospitalization charges not covered by their insurance because an unjustified test (ranging in cost from $81 to $620*) had been ordered, would they recall how aggressively *they* demanded this *pricey* test? Would an unfortunate billing representative who answered their call be tormented with wild claims against that doctor who should not have ordered a test he knew was unnecessary? Then, once the infuriated Manns finally gained the audience of hospital executives, would those executives, in response, seek out nurse Mark who had cautioned physician Benson to obey the parents? Or, would the executives instead yank Benson from his day to explain his weak rationale for ordering a test that has enraged the customer and has now cost the hospital considerably more than the cost of the test itself? Suddenly, despite his intentions to satisfy the customer, the nurse and Administration, Benson would have to defend himself from what he feared most – trouble with administrative involvement.

Although the act to stand one's ground and not order the test seems to be the better decision, it too would have repercussions. Mr. and Mrs. Mann could have been relishing the chance to diagnose their daughter when the doctor could not; they could have ignored little Miss Mann's daily improvement, focusing solely on Benson's insubordination; and could have hounded Administration with the "customer is always right" truism. Depending on Administration's priority – ratings versus profit – Benson could have found himself either berated or backed by the administrators.

Seemingly a lose-lose situation, Benson must ultimately decide which course of action would be personally acceptable. Given the fickle nature of the human ego and perspective, either decision would be a gamble. Now litigiously sensible, the next time Benson grapples between a Mann or the industry standards, he may want to arm himself with medical doctrines. (Maybe then he can have at least one standing leg if or when a dispute erupts.)

*Based on the 2013 APHL-CDC Influenza Cost Estimation Models.
https://www.aphl.org/programs/infectious_disease/influenza/Documents/ID_2013Sept_APHL-CDC-Influeza-Cost-Estimation-Models.pdf

if it walks like a duck …

A staggering 42-year-old Mr. Mann complained of abdominal pain and nausea. He confessed to binging on alcohol. The ER course confirmed Mr. Mann's greatly intoxicated state; his impressively elevated blood alcohol level corroborated Mr. Mann's story. A CAT scan of the abdomen had no concerning findings. Still, his discomfort persisted despite several doses of IV analgesics. Hospitalist Bill was asked to admit Mr. Mann. Bill concluded that the belly pain was likely acute gastritis from the alcohol. In severe and extreme cases, stomach lining irritation, or gastritis, can cause ulcers and internal bleeding. Oftentimes, however, the gastritis symptoms improve after a brief period of bowel rest, during which the individual does not eat but receives IV fluids for hydration, antacids, and IV analgesics. With that in mind, Bill decided an overnight hospital stay for these treatments would alleviate Mr. Mann's symptoms.

Bill also noticed the gentleman's gait was quite unsteady. He consulted Neurology to evaluate this ataxia (loss of full control of bodily movements). He signed off his plans to fellow hospitalist Finn, who would be Mr. Mann's attending physician.

As predicted, Mr. Mann's symptoms improved the following day. His abdominal pain resolved completely. He was ready to eat again. Finn ordered a light, bland breakfast as a slow, easy start for the recovering stomach. By lunch, Finn graduated the diet to a regular, solid meal. Mr. Mann tolerated both very well. Finn concluded that Mr. Mann was safe for discharge home following review of medical recommendations for alcohol cessation and information for outpatient resources. He thoroughly reexamined the gentleman before formally discharging him home without the neurology consult.

Mr. Mann had no transportation home. Finn offered arrangements for transportation by the social worker. Mr. Mann declined, stating that he lives only six miles away and preferred to walk home "for the exercise." As he watched a sober Mr. Mann stride steadily out of the hospital, Finn wondered how that neurology consult would have benefited this man who just could not walk steadily while drunk.

■ ■ ■

How does that saying go?
– If he talks like a drunk, smells like a drunk, staggers like a drunk, then he's just drunk.

Or maybe it's about quacking, waddling and a duck. Either way, if all clinical signs undoubtedly point in one direction, why stagger down the opposite?

doctoring a myth

A 31-year-old Mr. Mann presented with joint pains in his lower back and hips. He said the pain was typical for his sickle cell anemia. As a homeless man living in his car and having recently moved to California from Louisiana, he had not yet established a primary physician prior to finishing his medications.

Routine treatment of sickle cell crisis* consists of IV fluids and IV narcotics. Hospitalist Luis treated Mr. Mann accordingly while awaiting prior medical records from Louisiana. Luis consulted hematologist Phillip for collaborative care. Phillip noticed Mr. Mann's current blood work was not typical for sickle cell disease; he then ordered a hemoglobin electrophoresis diagnostic test that distinguishes the type of sickle cell anemia. There are two types: sickle cell disease and sickle cell trait. People prone to sickle cell crisis have sickle cell disease; those who have sickle cell trait are carriers that can pass the gene for sickle cell disease to their offspring but do not suffer from crises. Mr. Mann's hemoglobin electrophoresis confirmed sickle cell TRAIT. Phillip documented his findings and signed off the case. Phillip never discussed the test results with Mr. Mann.

Nevertheless, Mr. Mann remained in the hospital receiving IV fluids and narcotics daily for his complaints documented as "sickle cell pain crisis." The IV narcotics were ordered PRN or "as needed" every two hours. Without fail, every two hours, Mr. Mann reported pain, received narcotics and promptly departed the hospital to sit in his car for two hours, returning just in time for his next dose. He refused the therapeutic IV fluids and accepted only the IV narcotics to treat his illness. Such was his way until hospital day six when hospitalist Art signed on to the service.

Art informed Mr. Mann that, as per usual care for sickle cell crisis, the narcotics would be weaned off in the absence of discomfort. Mr. Mann objected to stopping his well-established two-hour narcotic pushes. Noticing that the Louisiana medical records had not arrived, Art then insisted Mr. Mann provide the name of his former medical provider. Mr. Mann reluctantly voiced a name then refused to answer any other questions. Art asked the ward secretary to check for local medical records in addition to records from the provider Mr. Mann named. The following day, Art sifted through ten different hospital records successfully retrieved throughout the region. Mr. Mann had been treated in either a hospital or an emergency room for "sickle cell crisis" and discharged with a prescription for narcotics ten times within a span of just three weeks!

Coincidentally, Mr. Mann informed the nursing staff that he would leave the hospital unless he was assigned another hospitalist. When told there was no indication to reassign doctors, he walked out of the hospital against medical advice and never returned.

...

Clearly a case of hush 'em up, keep 'em calm, give 'em whatever, then run – er – sign off service.

With shifty characters like Mr. Mann, pacifying the patient until one's stint is over has become many hospitalists' method. Self-preservation is a necessary evil in bustling occupations; but self-preservation to avoid conflict is cowardly. The repercussions of cowardice affects *everything* and *everyone*.

Start with *Everything*:

Once Mr. Mann's lie had been unveiled by the hemoglobin electrophoresis test, plans to remove him from the facility needed to be accomplished quickly. A bed, at least one IV catheter, several meals, cups for drinking, hospital gowns, water for toilet flushes plus showers, electricity for lighting, and electricity for the television are expenses that should be provided for acutely ill patients with confirmed disease. In addition, when emergency departments frantically shift to an overflow status and await availability of beds, the Mr. Manns of the hospital boldly stroll to and from their beds and await their next fix – er – prescribed dose of narcotics.

Now consider *Everyone*:

The nurses bear the brunt of this waste of time, training and expense. They are tasked to be dedicated drug footmen for Mr. Mann. Anticipate the confrontation that would occur each time the nurses were unable to deliver the drug precisely when expected. Predict the unrest Mr. Mann would cause if anyone dared to challenge his request by reassessing his pain level or offering a lower dose. In addition to the one-on-one interactions, the nurses must endure Mr. Mann's antics during daily collaborative rounds. Fortunately, during such rounds, the antics are generously distributed among physician(s), case managers, therapists, and other team members whose time and talents could serve someone acutely ill with real disease.

Hospitalist Luis appeared to have prized his self-preservation over all else by jotting down notes until he could safely rid *himself* of responsibility. Art's actions, too, show an appreciation for his own self-preservation; he chose not to challenge Mr. Mann's lie with the results of the hemoglobin test. Instead, he saved himself from a fiery conversation. Yet, Art also chose not to humor Mr. Mann's habit. By shielding his treatment plan (to lessen then stop the drugging) behind industry standards, Art gained control of Mr. Mann's care. Art strengthened his stance against Mr. Mann's abuse of the system by pressing the team to find other providers and any local records. With undeniable evidence revealing Mr. Mann's lying (the hemoglobin test) and drug-seeking behaviors (the ten other medical visits for narcotics), the rest of the medical team was empowered to deny his request to change doctors.

Although the mistreatment of a lie is largely the fault of the hospitalist, there are two accomplices that share blame – the hematologist and the hospital policy:

Hematologist Phillip had immediately detected the falsehood, so he appropriately ordered a diagnostic study to prove his suspicions correct. Confirming that no sickle cell disease and, thus, no related crisis existed, Phillip prematurely terminated his services by failing to inform Mr. Mann about the test results. Sure, Phillip had no therapeutic interventions to offer; but he had an ethical obligation to "inform" Mr. Mann that his type of sickle cell does not cause crisis. The hospitalist needed to resolve his narcotic abuses and discharge him; Phillip only needed to report his findings to the patient. Had he done so, Phillip may have empowered the first hospitalist, Luis, to stop Mr. Mann's deceits. Or, Phillip's report could have flustered Mr. Mann, who could have felt exposed, feared the consequences and bolted from the hospital. Having not been confronted, Mr. Mann returned every two hours for his narcotics. In fact, he routinely left the hospital floor, the building and quite possibly the parking lot between doses. It was as if he had been blessed with a free, at will pharmacy gifting nightly lodging. Had the hospital enforced a policy restricting floor departures or provided closely monitored off-floor areas within the facility, Mr. Mann may not have lingered for long.

Notwithstanding the lack of collaboration from Phillip and the lack of enforcement from hospital policy, it is the hospitalist who must flex his power to achieve honest medicine. When all others fail, the hospitalist needs to succeed. The collective welfare depends on it.

* During a sickle cell crisis, the red blood cells change from a round shape into a sticky crescent (or sickle) then clump together in various vessels throughout the body. This clumping of sickled red blood cells stops blood flow and compromises the supply of oxygen and needed nutrients. Consequently, sufferers experience excruciating pain, most frequently in the limbs, joints and chest. Controlling this crisis requires aggressive intravenous hydration, pain control and, if severe, supplemental oxygen. Failure to provide sufficient hydration will result in worsening crisis that becomes life-threatening due to compromised blood circulation to vital organs.

yep, they call us Doctor!

"The art of medicine consists of amusing the patient while nature cures the disease." Voltaire

- An elderly woman presented with stroke symptoms. The head CAT scan ruled out brain hemorrhage. Still, there was concern for ischemia, lack of blood flow. Probable ischemia, which could lead to more aggressive, debilitating CVA (cerebral vascular accident), requires aspirin immediately until an MRI rules out stroke. *Eighteen hours later,* while awaiting the MRI results, the hospitalist had one question: What happened to the aspirin?! None was ordered.

  (Dear Body, thank you! The MRI was negative. Whew!)

- A 56-year-old man presented with intense back pain resulting in leg weakness; he could hardly walk. The CAT scan showed no fractures or other abnormalities. Concern for spinal cord compression led to an overnight observation, an MRI and the need for stat IV steroids. The MRI, completed first thing in the morning, confirmed vertebral herniations that were flattening the spinal cord. Upon receiving such frightening results, the hospitalist had one question: What happened to the steroids?! None was ordered.

  (Dear Body, thank you for keeping the swelling at bay; now this man will walk again.)

A little editing goes a long way …

- *Exact* transcription signed off by the hospitalist:

"... given the size of both her legs and swelling I suspect the patient is either occlusion or near occlusion filter. Term with this at the present time would allow a significant thrombus load to propagate forwards perhaps Toward her lungs. Little to do
In regard to her antilipid status is considered to be held finally got studies were also changed to every 6 hours coverage. May need to decrease the Lantus dose slightly."

- *Exact* transcription signed off by the hospitalist:
  "Patient's only complaint at present she's hurting. She admits she is hurting every since she has as I'm hurting in it. She does have a PCA pump running but I suspect she was quite anxious also. He denies chest pain. She denies shortness of breath. She denies"

Mullerian and Wolffian are not one and the same ...

- A patient presents to the ER. As part of routine work-up, the doctor orders a pregnancy test.
  The patient is a visibly ego syntonic, biological male.

- A patient presents to the ER. As part of routine work-up, the doctor orders a PSA (Prostate Specific Antigen) for his patient.
  The patient is a visibly ego syntonic, biological female.

Genius!

- *Exact* assessment – plan:
  "morbid obesity – remains obese"

- The hospitalist performs a complete history and physical exam on the patient. He introduces himself and inquires about the events leading to her admission. He raises only one eyebrow at her odd, inappropriate answers. Nevertheless, he concludes the visit, leaves the room then types his assessment. Finally, as he nearly finishes the orders, he launches both eyebrows to the roof – she was the wrong patient.

HOSPITALIST TO (SUB)SPECIALIST

i'm not your brain!

Admitting physician Whit reviewed his assessment and plan with fellow hospitalist Richard regarding a woman who had presented with shortness of breath due to severe anemia.

Several years prior, the woman elected to have gastric bypass surgery which resulted in poor absorption of nutrients, including iron. Poor nutrient absorption requires individuals to take nutritional supplements indefinitely. This person stopped all supplements in her diet, creating a severe iron-deficient state that led to life threatening anemia. She required blood and iron transfusions to boost her red blood cell count until daily oral iron supplements could support sufficient cell levels.

Richard nodded as he processed the information. Richard asked when Whit planned to call the hematologist. Confused, Whit slowly shook his head in response. The hospitalists concluded their exchange.

Richard consulted the hematologist for direction. The expert hematologist agreed that treatment with blood transfusion and intravenous iron during hospitalization followed by oral iron supplements upon discharge was all that was needed.

■ ■ ■

Once upon a time, the internist was the doctors' doctor. Internists managed straightforward cases on their own. Now and again, they would be stumped by a real *head-scratcher*, a *zebra*, an unusual cluster of signs and symptoms. If they did not know the diagnosis, they slimmed the possibilities to two or three. Then (and only then) would they seek a subspecialist. That time is not today.

Today, internists routinely consult specialists and rely on the consultants' notes for management. Now, internists insist on a pulmonary consult for uncomplicated pneumonia. Contemporary internists rely on nephrologists to resolve any suggestion of dehydration. Meanwhile, these very internists expect respect.

Returning to Richard, did he consider the hematologist's load? Richard knows conducting a history and physical for the simplest of cases can be time consuming. The internist appears to have taken the privilege of expert consulting for granted. In fact, an expert may interpret it as mockery.

Next, consider the burden placed upon the subspecialist: *I've been called to act; therefore, I must act … upon … something. …*

Fortunately, in this instance, the hematologist did not feel obligated to order unnecessary tests. In other cases, diagnostic tests are ordered when an uninformative or a negative yield is expected. What appears as a quick and simple request converts into excessive expenditures of resources, from physicians, nurses and supporting staff (phlebotomists, lab technicians, radiology technicians) to electrical energy, radiation exposures, biohazardous wastes, and so on.

Such seemingly casual requests suggest that the internist has become uneasy about managing medical matters. Or, rather, he would prefer someone think for him. This dependency on subspecialists undermines the respect, trust and faith from patients in his care. True, following someone else's lead is simpler than leading; but, Doctors, today is time to reclaim the skill internal medicine requires from the Internist.

In reverence of internist, Dr. Laurence (Larry) Feenstra – the quintessential doctors' doctor

i'm not your scribe!

Tucked in a hidden room within earshot of the nurses' station, internist Hunter logs his assessment and plan for the person he had last examined. Keeping one ear cocked, Hunter stays alert to the goings on outside his workroom. He overhears general surgeon Ben discussing a patient's discharge with the nurse.

Due to the hospital's recent conversion to a new electronic medical record system, Ben, who has not yet learned the system, exasperatedly informs the nurse that he will not complete the electronic discharge and asks the nurse to finish it. Unfamiliar with physician discharges, the nurse cannot complete Ben's discharge. In a flash, Ben has a brilliant idea:

"Consult the hospitalist!"

Slacked jaw and peeved, Hunter awaits the consult. Hunter then phones Ben to kindly demonstrate the discharge process using one of his own internal medicine patients as an example. Hunter relates that, like Ben's, his job is to care for patients and not complete someone else's errands.

. . .

Like seedy bathrooms, are there markings on operating room walls? Would hospitalists gasp at the site of their pager number scrawled beneath the words: "For a good scribe, call _____"?

Although Ben and Hunter's case illustrate patient-punting at the time of discharge, this also occurs during admissions. Patients with primarily surgical issues are routinely deferred to hospitalist services, allowing surgeons to skip alongside as "consultants."

Consulting physicians can swiftly see patients, handsomely bill for their services and basically avoid nurse calls or discharge procedures. Surgeons' most common argument centers on individuals with multiple medical problems. Of course, no one expects a surgeon to manage a web of pulmonary plus cardiac plus endocrine plus renal plus more and more chronic issues; hospitalists are more than willing to consult and stabilize chronic medical conditions, because, if they do not, these complex patients will crash.

Sure, clerical tasks burden doctors. Really, who wants to deal with that secretarial stuff? No one. Nevertheless, these tasks are part of the job. Unless one's physician network can afford a clerical service, everyone – hospitalists, surgeons and other disciplines alike – must be prepared to accept all responsibilities that rightfully belong to his service.

In addition, saddle the ego. One discipline is not greater than another. If that were the case, no interdisciplinary consulting would occur. Despite the sensational monetary disparity between procedural disciplines and nonprocedural disciplines, no one specialty bears the right to undermine another just because the other is not trained to accomplish the one's job.

In short, the problem is the solution: Respect and Responsibility.

Everyone deserves R&R.

enterprising consults for the Good ... or the Gold?

Pulmonology

A woman with chronic obstructive pulmonary disease (COPD) required hospitalization and treatment for her shortness of breath. Due to her dependence on supplemental oxygen despite standard treatment with intravenous steroids and bronchodilators, a pulmonologist assisted in her care. Within days, the woman's breathing eventually improved toward her norm.

Suddenly, right before she prepared to transition out of the hospital, she developed severe abdominal pain and further testing revealed that this was from a small bowel obstruction. In her remote past, she had a complex abdominal surgery that left scar tissue. Sometimes extensive intraabdominal scarring (adhesions) can block the normal flow of the small intestines creating a small bowel obstruction as had now occurred. She did not respond to intravenous fluids, pain medication, bowel rest and nasogastric suction. Instead, she required another abdominal surgery to break up the intestinal adhesions.

Given her prior abdominal surgery years before, this procedure was exceptionally difficult. Consequently, the woman remained hospitalized – her bowels stopped functioning for several weeks and all nutrition was administered intravenously as TPN or total parenteral nutrition.

Her initial pulmonary distress had completely resolved prior to the surgery weeks ago. Yet, day after day, the pulmonologist saw fit to see her faithfully then bill her for his dedication.

Cardiology

Following a frightening episode of rectal bleeding, a woman had been hospitalized to determine whether the episode signaled ongoing internal bleeding. She had a medical history of heart disease; but she did not suffer any symptoms related to her heart or lungs. She sailed through her brief two-day hospitalization with no further bleeding.

Nevertheless, her cardiologist heard about her hospitalization. Neither awaiting – let alone requesting – a formal consult nor following the practice of first conversing with the responsible hospitalist, the cardiologist flocked to the woman (especially her chart) and directly billed for his unsolicited attentions.

Neurology

An elderly gentleman had a change in his behavior: he had become increasingly disengaged then outright lethargic. Except for modest dehydration, tests for infections, toxic ingestions, metabolic abnormalities, brain abnormalities, and cardiac instability were negative. Out of ideas, the hospitalist asked the neurologist to see him.

While awaiting the neurologist's evaluation, the hospitalist scrutinized the gentleman's home medicines which revealed a number of sedating agents that had been prescribed by several different, unsuspecting doctors. In addition to the sedatives' collective interactions, dehydration prevented his flushing these medications out of his body. The accumulation and prolonged exposure of those sedatives led to the man's altered mental status.

After stopping of the medications and administration of IV fluids, the gentleman perked up. He quickly resumed his normal behaviors. Mystery solved and treated; the hospitalist phoned the neurologist with the good news:

> Hospitalist: ... We will be sending him home.
>
> Neurologist: No! Don't send him yet. I'm almost in the hospital. Let me see him first.

Hospitalist: But he is fine. A neurology work-up is no longer
                 necessary.

The neurologist insisted upon seeing him, ordered a MRI (which returned normal), billed for his services, and agreed that the patient was free to go home.

■ ■ ■

In each of these situations, the subspecialists were either not needed at all or not needed for their respective patients' entire hospital course. It is a guilty pleasure for a provider to see and bill patients that require little intervention. Unlike providers from independent (not employed by the hospital or a corporation) subspecialties, the hospitalists rarely gain directly from billing patients. As employees, hospitalists often receive incentives to document properly and minimize the duration of patients' stay; they do not capitalize on patient billing as richly as their employers or the independent practitioners.

Now, one could argue that these three subspecialists' primary concern was the well-being of the hospitalized. Sure, one could conclude that.

If so, how can one explain the monetary gain in such altruistic concern, especially when the amount of compensation is determined by the selfless subspecialist himself? Then again, must the selfless starve?

If the means are as noble as the gestures, may the good-intentioned fatten his belly. Here, however, it seems that even if the three subspecialists had not rewarded themselves for their respective consults, their bellies will still be well fed. Perhaps, some of their daily comforts would require minor adjustments, but they will indeed still eat.

Everyone must eat, the provided for and the providers alike. Those who seek medical care often have a hefty bill awaiting their return home: the entire hospitalization – from the building itself to the people maintaining it – can factor into patients' fees. Regarding providers, even if their input *is* necessary, any provider added to a patient's treatment will raise the cost of that hospitalization. Third party payors can be helpful after the deductible is paid. However, third party payors search for loopholes, and, once they find those holes, charge the provided for and the providers respectively. Patients haggle with insurance companies over unanticipated fees; healthcare organizations sic coders on physicians to change their documentation to something reimbursable.

Yes, everyone must eat; and no one eats for free. Be that as it may, should flattening another's belly justify any means to fatten one's own?

copy & go medicine

Mr. Mann presented with shortness of breath. He has cirrhosis, a severe liver disease that causes fluid retention throughout the body. After initial evaluation in the emergency department, Mr. Mann's breathing difficulties revealed fluid accumulation in his lung sac, known as pleural effusion. Hospitalist Andy admitted Mr. Mann, consulted gastroenterologist Greg for further management, then submitted his admitting assessment and plan. Greg was not available; Andy instead consulted gastroenterologist Chester. Both Andy and Chester separately completed their required documentation.

Hospitalist Andy's Admission Note:

HISTORY OF PRESENT ILLNESS:

Mr. Mann is a 78-year-old man with shortness of breath for one week, worse with exertion walking across a room. No chest pain. Had some abdominal pain prior to thoracentesis. Has dry cough. No fever/chills. Nausea, but no emesis. Admitted one month ago and had thoracentesis. Has appointment with GI Dr. Greg but has not seen him yet. Dark stools one week ago but have not recurred. Reports water pill stopped by kidney doctor one week ago as it was not working well. Thoracentesis done today with 2.5L removed.

ASSESMENT AND PLAN:

Cryptogenic cirrhosis with ascites – previous admission. Call Dr. Greg, GI, in AM. Patient is supposed to see him as an outpatient soon, was deemed not good candidate for liver biopsy. Paracentesis ordered for 5/29. 2g sodium diet, check daily weights, fluid restrict.

Right Pleural Effusion – likely hepatic hydrothorax. 2.5L removed by thoracentesis 5/28. Chest x-ray procedure without pneumothorax. On room air.

Gastroenterologist Chester's Consultation Note:

HISTORY OF PRESENT ILLNESS:

Mr. Mann is a 78-year-old man with shortness of breath for one week, worse with exertion walking across a room. No chest pain. Had some abdominal pain prior to thoracentesis. Has dry cough. No fever/chills. Nausea, but no emesis. Admitted one month ago and had thoracentesis. Has appointment with GI Dr. Greg but has not seen him yet. Dark stools one week ago but have not recurred. Reports water pill stopped by kidney doctor one week ago as it was not working well. Thoracentesis done today with 2.5L removed. Cryptogenic cirrhosis with ascites – previous admission. Call Dr. Greg, GI, in AM. Patient is supposed to see him as an outpatient soon, was deemed not good candidate for liver biopsy. Paracentesis ordered for 5/29. 2g sodium diet, check daily weights, fluid restrict.

Right Pleural Effusion – likely hepatic hydrothorax. 2.5L removed by thoracentesis 5/28. Chest x-ray procedure without pneumothorax. On room air.

Hospitalist Andy's Admission Note:
(Continued)

Gastroenterologist Chester's Consultation Note:
(Continued)

Acute Kidney Injury – Pre-renal with hypervolemia versus hepatorenal. Check urinalysis. Give 40mg IV Lasix and albumin bolus. Check urine studies, renal ultrasound.

Acute Kidney Injury – Pre-renal with hypervolemia versus hepatorenal. Check urinalysis. Give 40mg IV Lasix and albumin bolus. Check urine studies, renal ultrasound.

Thrombocytopenia and coagulopathy – likely from liver disease.

Thrombocytopenia and coagulopathy – likely from liver disease.

Osteoarthritis, chronic back pain – Minimize Tylenol. Will change to oxycodone. IV morphine as needed for pain.

Osteoarthritis, chronic back pain – Minimize Tylenol. Will change to oxycodone. IV morphine as needed for pain.

Lactic Acidosis – No evidence of infection. Do not repeat test for lactic acid.

Lactic Acidosis – No evidence of infection. Do not repeat test for lactic acid.

Black stools one week ago – Check stool for occult blood. IV PPI.

Black stools one week ago – Check stool for occult blood. IV PPI.

Prophylaxis: GI – PPI, DVT – mechanical intervention, plan paracentesis tomorrow

Prophylaxis: GI – PPI, DVT – mechanical intervention, plan paracentesis tomorrow

Diet: NPO start now

Diet: NPO start now

Fluid restriction 1500 mL's per day

Fluid restriction 1500 mL's per day

Mobility: as tolerated

Mobility: as tolerated

Code Status: Full

Code Status: Full

ASSESSMENT AND PLAN: check stool for occult blood. Watch CBC, ammonia. May be a candidate for TIPS or porto-venous shunt. If stool occult blood is positive, will do endoscopy early next week.

. . .

Plainly, gastroenterologist Chester so carelessly copied hospitalist Andy's admission note that his "History of Present Illness" makes no sense! Did gastroenterologist Chester truly intend to consult gastroenterologist Greg too? Since when did a gastroenterologist tackle kidney issues or chronic back pain? Given the inconsistencies in his note, one must wonder whether Chester actually evaluated the patient before simply tossing habitual phrases into the assessment and plan just to complete his documentation – or, rather, personalize his plagiarism.

anyone for a buck, eh?

DIVERTICULOSIS:

In diverticulosis, pockets (diverticula) develop in the intestinal wall. These pockets are fragile, with a tendency to bleed. Rarely, the bleeding can be persistent and life threatening. Commonly, the bleeding is brief and self-limited. Only during massive, uncontrollable bleeding is surgical removal of the affected bowel section recommended. In most cases, the bleeding stops without intervention. Once bleeding stops, patients are advised to maintain healthy fiber and fluid intake to ensure soft, regular bowel movements. (Retained constipated stool aggravates the fragile bowel wall.)

A rather independent 99-year-old Ms. Mann recently resettled to live with her adult children, who assisted her with more complex chores and tasks. She presented to the hospital immediately after an episode of bright red bleeding from her rectum. The bleeding stopped as instantly as it started. Gastroenterologist Brayden scheduled a colonoscopy for the next day.

Hospitalist Riley, who assessed Ms. Mann the day after admission, concluded that the brief, transient bleeding from her rectum resulted from either diverticulosis or internal hemorrhoids. Her labs showed stable hemoglobin levels that did not require transfusions or other interventions. Riley weighed Ms. Mann's baseline condition. She was a fairly healthy 99-year-old, but even the simplest invasive procedure could compromise her elderly state; it could perforate her thinned bowel wall. Or, the sedation could be her downfall, tipping her into a delirium that cascades into lethal outcomes. Her bleeding had stopped on its own. Riley concluded the risks exceeded the benefits. He discussed his assessment with Brayden.

Riley: Ms. Mann looks good and is no longer bleeding. I think that it's best that we discharge her and have her follow up with her primary care doctor regularly.

Brayden: She agrees to get a colonoscopy first.

Riley: She just told me that she agreed to get the colonoscopy, because you told her she needed one. In fact, she specifically said, "I'll do whatever the doctor says I should do."

Brayden: So, you don't want me to do the colonoscopy?

Riley: The bleeding seems diverticular or, perhaps, hemorrhoidal. And now it's stopped. What exactly are you looking for in this colonoscopy?

Brayden: What if she has cancer that made her bleed?

Riley: Even if she had cancer, what would we do about it?

Brayden: Well, we just have to see. We can discuss that when we get there.

Riley: She's 99 years old! Nobody is going to do anything about cancer in a 99-year-old. The treatment for the cancer would be worse than naturally dying from the cancer. I feel that, in the absence of any recurrent bleeding, in this mature woman, we should do our due diligence in educating her and leave well enough alone.

Brayden: Well, if you don't want me to do a colonoscopy, I won't do it. I'm always here to do my job. Let me know when you need me.

■ ■ ■

According to the Medscape Gastroenterologist Compensation Report 2019, at a $417K average income, "Gastroenterologists are among the top earners of all physician specialties." (Leslie Kane, MA | April 24, 2019)

The Colonoscopy Center for Excellence in San Francisco, California advertised that one of their cost advantages is a 46% lower cost than the average. With that advantage, a person with no insurance can anticipate the following fees:

>Colonoscopy Center's facility fee: Colonoscopy $1,492.
>
>Colonoscopy with biopsy and/or polyp (one or more) removal: $1,620
>
>Gastroenterologist fee: $500
>
>Anesthesiologist fee: $240
>
>Pathology fee: this depends on the number of polyps removed. You will receive a separate bill from the Pathology Department at California Pacific Medical Center. If no polyps are removed, there will be no Pathology fee.
>
>Clinical Laboratory fee: this will only apply if your physician took stool samples
>(https://www.sanfranciscocolonoscopy.com/about-colonoscopy/colonoscopy-cost/)

So, Dr. Brayden, in all honesty, was it really about cancer?

inconvenient medicine

Ms. Mann, a spry 70-year-old woman, went to the emergency room complaining about intermittent chest pain over the past four weeks. The pain felt like a dull pressure on the left side of her chest, which seemed to come and go unpredictably. She considered herself active, walking and occasionally running several days a week; so, this chest pain worried her. She had family members suffering active heart disease and was concerned that she, too, may have heart disease.

Hospitalist Trent, once he concluded that cardiovascular or pulmonary damage was unlikely, deduced that her symptoms likely stemmed from anxiety about the radical changes in her family's cardiac health. Still, at her age, Trent decided a cardiac stress test to assess impaired circulation was sensible. Given her active lifestyle, he confirmed with Ms. Mann that she would be able to run on a treadmill for this test.

Trent later followed up on the test results. Trent saw that the treadmill stress test had been switched to a chemical stress test. Chemical stress tests are designed for individuals who are not physically able to exert themselves. Ms. Mann confidently stated that she could run on a treadmill; the staff made no effort to attempt this noninvasive method prior to proceeding with the chemical alternative.

Perplexed, Trent contacted the overseeing cardiologist Ron:

Ron: The stress lab technician was concerned that a 70-year-old was going to run a treadmill, so he asked me to change it to a chemical stress test since she's old.

Trent: But we know there's no age limit to physical capability, and this patient is a lifelong runner and is very fit.

Ron: It's okay. I agree with you. I just went ahead and changed the test; because otherwise they'll keep calling me until they get what they want.

Trent, realizing his appeals were ringing in finger-clogged ears, relented. He sat annoyed that an exceptionally fit woman would be forced to introduce a useless chemical into her robust body solely to appease a technician. As Trent expected, the chemical stress test returned superbly normal. In fact, Ms. Mann's heart rivaled that of a healthy 35-year-old's. She was discharged home with a *clean bill of health* and with suggestions for managing her life stressors.

...

The technician seemed determined to execute the most fitting test ... but ... for whom? While a treadmill cardiac stress test exerts the patient, it, in kind, exerts the administrator who must do more than inject a substance in a patient lying still the entire time. The treadmill demands higher levels of administrator-patient interaction and monitoring. Unlike the treadmill, a simple chemical injection permits one to cast glances to and from the screen then the patient until the timer completes the exam. Seriously, why must one work at work?

Cardiologist Ron may not believe that, but he did nothing to challenge it. Rather, he sought to continue his work unbothered. Based on the technician's and Ron's actions, it appears that the best test for this healthy woman was the option that lets one best rest. That way, the technician would not have to exert himself during the test, and Ron would not have to exert his patience fielding pages throughout the test.

Well, good for *them*.

divided we fall ... and for what?!

Mr. Mann, a reasonably healthy 40-year-old male, complained of shortness of breath. Tests revealed pneumonia on a chest x-ray. His heart was in excellent health. He was admitted to the hospital and cared for by hospitalist Parker, pulmonologist Chuck and cardiologist Lyle.

Despite improvement with antibiotics commonly recommended for uncomplicated pneumonia, Mr. Mann asked for more testing. Chuck obliged with a chest CAT scan in search of pulmonary blood clots. Negative for clots, the CAT scan just confirmed the pneumonia. Also, despite effective treatment with the current antibiotic regimen (which causes fewer side effects and lower chances for bacterial resistance), Mr. Mann had Chuck switch his antibiotics to a much more powerful combination.

Not quite content with the correct diagnosis, unnecessary testing, overly aggressive medications and improved breathing, Mr. Mann asked that even more testing be ordered to rule out other causes for his resolved breathing difficulties. He told Lyle, the cardiologist, to investigate his condition further. Lyle, certain that Mr. Mann's cardiac function was normal given normal cardiac enzymes and echocardiogram, conducted a stress test, which confirmed Mr. Mann's normal cardiovascular function.

Mr. Mann exceeded the typical hospital duration for a reasonably healthy male with uncomplicated pneumonia and continued to improve with IV antibiotic treatments. He had no fever, shortness of breath, poor oxygenation or elevated white blood cell counts. Based on standard practice, he could now transition to oral antibiotics and complete them at home. Hospitalist Parker addressed Mr. Mann's progress and advancement toward discharge. Not quite convinced, Mr. Mann *felt* he needed more days of intravenous antibiotics and convinced Chuck, the pulmonologist, to agree. In addition, Mr. Mann *felt* a cardiac angiogram must be completed prior to discharge. Wary, hospitalist Parker relayed the request to cardiologist Lyle. Both Parker and Lyle considered the test unnecessary. Parker mentioned that Mr. Mann was still wearing the cardiac monitor since admission seven days ago. The monitor recorded normal activity each day. Lyle agreed that the monitor could be discontinued.

Later that day, Mr. Mann asked the nurse to resume the cardiac monitor. Nurse Boyd paged Parker, who explained that both the cardiologist and he determined cardiac monitoring unnecessary at this point. Mr. Mann insisted the monitor be resumed. Boyd then paged cardiologist Lyle, who subsequently ordered the resumption of the cardiac monitor. Concurrently, pulmonologist Chuck obliged Mr. Mann's desire to remain hospitalized on IV antibiotics.

The following day, Parker approached Chuck about Mr. Mann's insistence for IV treatments and extended hospitalization despite medical readiness for discharge. Chuck agreed that Mr. Mann was stable to go home. Parker asked Chuck to join him in discussing the discharge plan with Mr. Mann.

At the sight of Parker, Mr. Mann verbally assaulted "the one who dared to stop his monitor the day before and now dared to conspire his discharge." Promptly, Parker was removed from Mr. Mann's *care* team.

Following Mr. Mann's eventual discharge, Boyd and other nurses confessed Mr. Mann stated that he did not want to return to work "too soon," and that "I plan to stay here for at least thirty days."

Note: The average hospital stay for pneumonia in the US is 5.4 days. Mr. Mann stretched his to ten.

■ ■ ■

Measly riggings in Mr. Mann's manipulations were these three physicians. Had Parker, Chuck and Lyle huddled backs-to-backs armed with stethoscopes in front, they could have defeated wasteful monitoring, testing, medicating and malingering. Alas, the three crumpled before the secondary gains of Mr. Mann and the well-played ploy of a nurse pleasing a demanding patient.

Like most indulged young children, Mr. Mann knew "the squeaky wheel gets the grease." Through relentless objections, Mr. Mann swayed two physicians to defy standard medical practice. This does not imply that Chuck and Lyle gained nothing. By ordering or conducting Mr. Mann's procedures, both physicians could capitalize by increasing their billing level. Chuck and Lyle also gain revenue by "seeing" a patient that does not need to be seen. In other words, with Mr. Mann improving daily to the extent he no longer required acute care in the hospital, the need to conduct full assessments is negated. Those once ten- to fifteen-minute examinations now required only five or fewer minutes.

Also, the number of disruptions from nurses campaigning for Mr. Mann decreased considerably when he was obeyed. By weakening their resolve, Chuck and Lyle became pawns for Boyd and other attendants. When nurse Boyd failed to obtain the order from hospitalist Parker, he straightaway dialed cardiologist Lyle. In an instant, obedient Lyle reduced physician authority to a scribe relaying the commands of Mr. Mann and Boyd.

This degradation could have been avoided had all three physicians acted jointly. Regardless of their distinct disciplines, the physicians are teammates with a united oath: heal or restore those in need through honest medicine. Failure to unite as a team and enforce honest practices is the ruin of medical integrity. Unjustifiable procedures and protracted hospital courses are vectors of ignoble healthcare. All three physicians needed to refuse Mr. Mann's demands. That means each physician must endure the ranting from Mr. Mann and the hounding from Boyd. In turn, like children, Mr. Mann will learn to mind medical boundaries and, in turn, stop hassling Boyd who, in turn, will stop hassling the physicians. Conversely, a disgruntled Mr. Mann will storm off AMA (against medical advice), shouting feeble threats as he discharges himself.

The lack of communication and commitment to an agreed care plan is not the fault of only Chuck and Lyle. Although Parker was trying to "do the right thing," as the hospitalist and the coordinating physician, he failed to unify the team. Parker had the added responsibility to hold the team accountable for acting in the best interest of the patient. He could not control the actions of his teammates, but he could keep them aware of the consequences. With respect and diplomacy, Parker could have continually redirected his colleagues toward the goal. Now, this does not make Parker an altruistic martyr by any means. No, he must protect his own hide when Administration tallies the number of protracted hospital stays and the number of these instances occurring each fiscal year. As the admitting and discharging physician for every instance, Parker will be the provider to blame for failure to meet hospital goals.

If only the three had banded together, then Chuck would not have surrendered to inapt practices, Lyle would not have been trivialized to a tool, and Parker would not have appeared inept in the timely management of uncomplicated pneumonia.

HOSPITALIST TO EMERGENCY PHYSICIAN

for the good of whom, again?

A middle-aged Ms. Mann with a history of chronic congestive heart failure presented to the ED complaining of worsening back pain. On this day, her chronic back pain suddenly intensified when she bent down to retrieve an object from the floor. In the ED, she received intravenous analgesics. Ned, the emergency physician, heard wheezing during his physical exam then ordered a chest x-ray. The x-ray illustrated fluid congestion. Ned phoned hospitalist Courtney to admit Ms. Mann for an exacerbation of congestive heart failure (CHF).

Courtney acknowledged that wheezing could occur during a CHF exacerbation, but it is not commonly the presenting symptom. He also noted that Ms. Mann's BNP (brain natriuretic peptide) level was quite low (~50 pg/mL), whereas in fulminant congestive heart failure, the BNP would be at least 300.

"Why do you feel that she needs to be admitted?" inquired Courtney.

"Because she has congestion on her chest x-ray," concluded Ned.

"But some people can have chronic congestion on their x-ray and not necessarily have distressing symptoms. Is she short of breath?"

"Well, she said she was wheezing. Er, yes, she is short of breath."

When Courtney interviewed Ms. Mann, she emphasized that only her back pain prompted her to seek help.

"Well the ED called me to admit you because they were concerned about your breathing," explained Courtney.

"My breathing?!" Ms. Mann questioned incredulously. "I feel fine. Matter of fact, this is better than usual!" She further explained how she uses oxygen with inhalers at home for her "lung disease" (COPD, chronic obstructive pulmonary disease) and that she "wheezes all the time." Indeed, on examination, Ms. Mann showed no signs of distress or acute breathing difficulties.

"I feel better now after that medicine they gave me for my back," Ms. Mann concluded.

"Well, you certainly look well and don't need to remain in the hospital."

"Thanks, doc! By the way, those sure are some nice shoes you have there!"

■ ■ ■

So, when the patient feels better and reports resolution of her presenting problem, one should admit her anyway? Hmm…

It is difficult to understand Ned's reasoning when Ms. Mann no longer has any complaints. Yes, her chest x-ray is not ideal in an ideal world; but, in Ms. Mann's world, that portrait of her lungs may have been a masterpiece given her *better-than-usual* breathing. Ned's reaction to a chest x-ray inspires a number of uncertainties:

Did he ask Ms. Mann if she had chronic lung disease during his history taking?

Did he ask her what medications and treatments she uses at home?

Did he think to mention or ask her about the wheezing he heard during the exam?

Did he notice her breathing was not labored?

Did he check her oxygen saturation level to determine any cardiopulmonary compromise?

Did he check any other vital signs?

Did he not see the BNP level?

Did he not know the BNP level was normal?

Did he think the chest x-ray was more credible than Ms. Mann's relaxed state?

Did he confuse her with another patient who was indeed short of breath during his rebuttal to Courtney?

Did he honestly think she needed to be admitted?

Did he care?

chest pain: NOT the usual suspect

Emergency physician calls the hospitalist for admissions to rule out heart attack:

50-year-old with squeezing chest pain

A man in his fifties complained of chest pain that began after emptying a truckload of firewood. He did not experience this pain during exertion. Only after he stopped the activity did he notice a squeezing sensation along the front of his chest.

Diagnosis: Chest Pain due to Pectoral Muscle Spasms

40-year-old with left arm pain

A woman in her forties complained of chest pain felt along her left arm. She worked in a laundromat; her duties required reaching above her head to grab bundles of high hanging clothes. She said the upper part of her chest wall (near her shoulder deltoid muscle) hurts "whenever I move my arm like this," as she lifted and stretched her arm backwards.

Diagnosis: Chest Pain due to Muscle Strain from Overextension Injury

29-year-old with left-sided chest pain

A fit appearing, muscular man in his late twenties presented with excruciating left-sided chest pain. In the middle of the night he had rushed out of bed to comfort his screaming three-month-old baby. As it was dark, he slammed his left chest into the sharp corner of a dresser, sustaining a painful, arrestingly visible bruise. Ibuprofen and a muscle relaxer promptly relieved his discomfort.

Diagnosis: Chest Pain due to Blunt Trauma

60-year-old with general chest pain

A man in his sixties presented with centralized chest pain. The emergency physician asked the hospitalist to admit the gentleman for cardiac testing. The hospitalist asked why the gentleman came to the hospital. The man said he had suffered a motor vehicle collision the prior week resulting in a fractured sternum; he ran out of pain medications prescribed at the time and came to the emergency department in hopes of getting refills until his appointment to see his primary care physician again. The hospitalist examined the gentleman. Gentle pressure applied to the man's fractured sternum precisely reproduced the chest pain.

Diagnosis: Chest Pain due to Fractured Sternum

70-year-old with right-sided chest pain

A woman in her seventies presented to the emergency room with sharp pain on the right side of her chest. Her pain was constant and unremitting irrespective of activity. At the suggestion of right-sided cardiac pain, the hospitalist raised his eyebrows – apart from rare genetic conditions, the heart is generally located on the left. This woman had no such genetic variant. With his *eyes*, the hospitalist instantly diagnosed the problem.

Diagnosis: Chest Pain due to Shingles Rash

■ ■ ■

The words chest and pain are a worrisome couple. The greatest fears following that verbal pairing are life-threatening cardiovascular conditions or massive blood clots in the lungs. These fears seem to trigger demands for immediate cardiac evaluation. The trendy "chest pain work-up" typically entails twenty-four-hour heart rhythm monitoring, serial cardiac enzymes levels, and a stress test.

Imagine enduring all that fuss for a rash!

One or two questions revealed the obvious mildness of those five individuals' respective ailments. These ill-fated five were almost sentenced to a pricey (well beyond the thousands), restless (continual interruptions for procedures), blood-sucking (lab tests), physiologically exerting (stress test) overnight stay far from the comforts of their own homes.

Is fear of adverse outcomes the source spurring these aggravations? Or are there other variables lurking beneath this compulsion to blindly admit the words "chest pain" to the hospital? Possible variables include poor history taking, disinterest in figuring out the issue, the desire to clear the patient census by any means or tucking all *cases* away so that one may leave the minute his shift ends.

If poor history taking is the matter, one should reconsider his occupation. Since the first year in medical school, doctors are conditioned to begin every evaluation with a patient history. In fact, compensated documentation requires not only the reasons the person presented to the hospital but also past medical conditions, past surgeries, current medications, allergies, family medical history, a social history (recreation and habits), an occupational history, and a review of all body systems that may be completely unrelated to the ER visit. So, if all that information must be documented with each visit to the ER and reiterated in the written admission note, poor patient history taking translates into either incompetence or negligence.

Perhaps disinterest fuels this trend toward indiscriminate chest pain admissions. After all, these admissions do not drain the doctor's dollar *or* steal time away from his life *or* upset his emotions. Rather, the doctor's quality of life will continue unbothered regardless if someone else's is. This disinterest could be tagged the "couldn't-care-less-as-long-as-there's-my-check" healthcare. On the contrary, maybe there *is* interest: Maybe quickening lead times from the minute the patient walks through the door to the minute the provider transfers the patient from the emergency department are rewarded with financial paybacks. $hooing a patient along any pipeline in record time$ may ju$tify hospitalizing healthy people.

It is likely that none of those reasons is a factor. It could just be about punctuality. If one starts his shift on time, one should end his shift on time. He showed up; he "saw" patients; he treated them with something; he sent them somewhere…safely; he completed his documentation; he fulfilled his obligation. Having accomplished the chore of providing *care*, he now deserves to be released from his post precisely on the hour. Whether those patients were aptly treated does not much matter so long as they have been passed off by the end of his shift.

Shifting from those variables, return to fear: Fearing a life-threatening cardiac or pulmonary condition when facing the situations illustrated above can appear like heroic caution. However, acting out of fear in such cases translates into unheroic amateurism.

it's treat the Person NOT the Number, right?

Fifty-year-old Mr. Mann presented to the ED with chest pain complaints.

(Twelve months prior, he had been diagnosed with drug-induced congestive heart failure. Since then, he changed his lifestyle by stopping recreational drug use, losing weight and quitting smoking. A recent cardiac stress test confirmed he had regained normal cardiac circulation and function. He no longer required routine assessments by a cardiologist.)

Shortly after arriving to the ED, the chest pain completely resolved. All tests were either normal or unremarkable, including serial cardiac enzymes, which are 2 to 3 sets of blood tests checked six hours apart. If someone were suffering a heart attack, cardiac enzymes would rise after six hours.

The chest pain never recurred. In the absence of any life-threatening cardiac illness, the ED physician Truett decided Mr. Mann could be safely discharged home. Moments before releasing Mr. Mann, Truett ordered *just one more* test, a lipase level. The lipase level returned elevated. Truett paged hospitalist Keaton. High lipase levels often occur in pancreatitis; symptoms include nausea, vomiting, and excruciating abdominal pain worsened by eating. Keaton asked Truett if Mr. Mann had any of these symptoms to which Truett replied, "No, but I can't explain why his lipase is high."

Keaton conversed with and examined Mr. Mann then discharged him home. Elated to be released, Mr. Mann shared, "Tomorrow's my birthday!"

■ ■ ■

Fancy a birthday on a gurney all because of a random number, a trifle that has no bearing on your actual condition.

The body is constantly fluctuating and regulating itself to maintain balance. Truett caught only a snapshot of this phenomenon. He captured an isolated elevated lipase level in the absence of any signs or symptoms to require overnight observation, let alone a full hospital admission.

Because the second-to-second logic of the human body cannot always be explained, novices training in medicine are instructed to investigate a patient's entire clinical presentation before reacting to a solitary level. Lab results must be considered within context. Mr. Mann's presentation lacked signs of distress prior to Keaton's evaluation. Therefore, the lipase level was little more than a quirk at that time. Such findings confuse many practitioners.

Those drills for training physicians to "treat the patient and not the number" are invaluable reminders to avoid wasting resources – or someone's birthday, namely Mr. Mann's.

uhh ... just admit 'em

Cared for by her husband and daughter, 83-year-old Mrs. Mann presented to the ED for changes in her behavior.

In older adults, a change in behavior or mental status typically signals an underlying infection. Urinary tract infections (UTI) are one of the most common causes. Often, shortly after treatment starts, the mental capacity improves, and normal behavior resumes.

ED physician Rob ordered tests that confirmed a UTI and requested admission. Hospitalist Gordon asked if Mrs. Mann's vital signs were unstable. Rob reported that she did not have unstable blood pressures, heart rates, fever or abnormal labs. Apart from the behavioral changes, Mrs. Mann had no other distressing signs.

Gordon questioned, "This patient sounds stable: is there any reason why she couldn't be prescribed antibiotics and be discharged home?"

Rob replied, "I don't think the family would like that plan. I believe they want her to be admitted."

"We can't just admit a patient because that's what the family wants. There has to be a valid reason. I will evaluate the patient and get back to you."

Prior to meeting Mrs. Mann, Gordon reviewed her chart. Mrs. Mann had been hospitalized three weeks prior with a similar presentation in which her behavior gradually escalated to hallucinations and paranoia. During that hospitalization, searching for any evidence of stroke, an extensive evaluation consisted of brain imaging, cardiac ultrasound, carotid artery ultrasound. All studies were unremarkable. Her urine studies revealed a UTI, however. A neurologist concluded she had underlying dementia resulting in cognitive decline. As a result, the acute urinary tract infection provoked Mrs. Mann's behavioral changes. The neurologist prescribed Aricept to slow dementia progression. She was discharged with Aricept for dementia and antibiotics for UTI. The family was educated about dementia and its unfortunate progression. Having completed this chart review, a frustrated Gordon cynically concluded that he had been asked to admit a patient for dementia, a nonacute condition that did not justify hospitalization.

As Gordon approached Mrs. Mann's room, her daughter (also the healthcare advocate) greeted him outside.

"Hi. I'm Dr. Gordon, the hospitalist. I was asked by the ED to evaluate your mother for admission."

"Admission?! I don't want her admitted! I brought her here because I want antibiotics for her bladder infection and a refill of the Aricept. We haven't gotten a chance to see her own doctor yet. I know this is all her dementia, and she has a UTI again. If she's admitted, she will get more confused and agitated in the hospital. She's much safer at home."

Gordon turned and faced Rob, who was within earshot.

"I agree with her. Based on my review of the chart and her statement, I feel her mother can safely return home. Do you still think I need to evaluate her for admission?"

"No," replied Rob, who directly proceeded with Mrs. Mann's discharge home.

• • •

Exactly what did Rob do prior to calling Gordon for an admission?

Apart from dismissing normal labs and vital signs, Rob's assessment for hospitalization lacked an actual assessment. In fact, it seems to have lacked the most critical component of all assessments – a history, a discussion with Mrs. Mann's family to learn about the need for medical assistance. Gordon barely ventured beyond introductions before Mrs. Mann's daughter explained the obvious diagnosis, the required treatment plan and the appropriate disposition. Also, in his request for admission, Rob cautioned Gordon that the family desired hospitalization. Rob either confused patients or lied.

Maybe what matters most is to just send the patient somewhere ... and quick.

The fastest out is the out that requires just two clicks: the first on some note template, the second on the order set "Admit to Medicine."

– habitually practiced as "Make Some Other Guy Deal with This"

try these shoes on for size

Once the Emergency Department determines that a patient requires admission, a text message is sent to the hospitalist triage phone, alerting the admitting physician to call the ED to accept the patient. As soon as the emergency physician relays the information, he immediately relinquishes all patient responsibilities to the receiving hospitalist. So, the sooner the hospitalist personally assesses the patient, the safer the patient will be. Otherwise the hospitalist is completely liable for a patient he has not yet evaluated.

Shortly after the start of his evening admitting shift, hospitalist Dylan received a text message to the triage phone. He promptly called the ED and was connected to two doctors, each requesting an admission. Dylan reviewed both patients' charts prior to briskly entering the ED to assess them. In transit, another text message alerted him. Estimating that he would require roughly twenty minutes to assess these first admissions, Dylan messaged: "I will call back in 20 minutes."

Dylan evaluated both patients and, before sitting down to place orders to finalize their admissions, he called the ED. This time, he was connected to three emergency physicians who passed a total of five new admissions. He jotted the new patients' names and locations then completed admission orders on the first two patients he had seen. Having conducted three conversations for new admissions and composing comprehensive order sets for two patients within forty-five minutes, Dylan reviewed the charts for his next five admissions then proceeded to assess them. Seconds before entering the first room, another text message alerted him. Calculating the time needed to assess these five patients, he messaged: "I will call back in 1 hour."

Dylan successfully completed his second (of five) assessments 18 minutes since his last text alert. Another message from the ED alerted him to call right away for additional admissions. Annoyed that he had not had the opportunity to see the three remaining patients, Dylan replied, "I will call back as soon as I can. I want to finish seeing these five." He hurriedly evaluated those remaining three, and the instant he sat before a computer, he received two pages from two different medical wards. He resolved the issues for the patients with their respective nurses. Reorienting his thoughts to the ED's agenda, Dylan breathed. Right then, ED director Henry entered the documentation room.

Henry: My ER doctors have been waiting for you to call back for the past hour.

Dylan: Yes, I know. I had to see the five new admissions that I already had pending.

Henry: I've talked to your boss about this before. I can't have my doctors waiting an hour to give you new admissions. I have a doctor that's been ready to go home but has had to wait for you for the past hour.

Dylan: He can pass the info to the next ED doc. I received seven admissions within two hours. I need to make sure those patients are safely secured before taking on more admissions. I'm asking that your doctors share this burden and continue caring for those patients until I can safely take more.

Henry: My doctors do not need to wait for an hour before talking to you.

Dylan: I will not take on more admissions until I make sure these five
are safe. I will call back in a few minutes.

Irritated, Dylan called the ED. Once again connected to three doctors, Dylan jotted down three new admissions, one from each emergency physician. So now, in the span of three hours, the hospitalist was charged with *10* admissions! Before he could place orders on the five earlier admissions prior to his latest batch, a nurse paged Dylan to address an issue for one of his pending admissions.

Sighing, Dylan reflected: First, he was expected to oversee more than 75 people already hospitalized, any of whom could have a crisis at any moment. Second, as the sole hospitalist on evening duty, he was responsible for accepting admission requests from several different emergency physicians, all of which have occurred simultaneously. Third, he must call back instantly every time a new request alerted his pager, regardless if he had a chance to see the earlier ones. Fourth, once the ED passed off the pending admissions, Dylan was wholly responsible for them. That means, if anyone crashes before Dylan could evaluate him, Dylan would be liable because he accepted a phone call.

"How is this safe?!" grumbled Dylan.

Dylan worked as swiftly and as diligently as his mortality permitted. By the end of his ten-hour shift, Dylan blazed through nine admissions, passing three on to the incoming admitting hospitalist. On his way home. Dylan kept mulling over details he may have missed during all that hustling.

"How could I ever, in good conscience, send my family to something like this?!"

· · ·

Considering the expected time spent on one typical, level 3 hospital admission is 70 minutes, Dylan's request for an hour to safely admit five people does not seem terribly unreasonable. Then again, if the emergency department follows Samuel Shem's *House of God*, any obstructions to immediate ejection of patients from the emergency room cannot be tolerated. Shem's portrait of the emergency room validates director Henry's anger with Dylan. Dylan should have disregarded his lengthy list of sick patients awaiting care so that he could accept punts from healthy physicians who want to go home.

So, why should the healthy not be liberated from their post after a grueling shift?

So, why could the emergency physicians not have done what all other specialties do when one's time is finished? They knew how to pass patients to other specialties. Their director, Henry, could have easily coordinated transition of care, had he prioritized patient safety. Instead, Henry prioritized clearing his docs' dockets by shifting responsibility to the opponent – pardon – the hospitalist. As the director who deals with the bigger picture, Henry should have worked with the sole hospitalist for the best outcome for the patients. Or, being an administrator, he could have worked with Dylan to ensure the best statistics for the hospital network by preventing morbidities (or, worse, fatalities) due to physician burnout. Henry could have seen this situation as a team crisis, not an *us-versus-him* clash.

Henry's anger about his footmen's predicament is understandable. However, his fight is not with the opposing footman, the hospitalist; his scuffle belongs on the administrative front. Administration should know the volume of patients its ED manages. Administration would be the entity that would effectively resolve conflicts or obstructions to patient care. Administration could find the funds necessary to prevent a ganging of five emergency physicians on one hospitalist by leveling the playing field with a proportionate number of hospitalists. Rather than misplace his anger, Henry should think of first, protecting the patients; second, advocating for his ED subordinates; then third, redressing the rightful offender behind the ED-Hospitalist row – The System.

wording then rewording 'til they admit

Ms. Mann presents to the emergency room with abdominal pain. Evaluation in the emergency department (ED) consists of a CAT scan negative for any abnormalities and laboratory studies revealing an elevated calcium level. Although the woman's abdominal pain resolves, the overseeing emergency physician Tom calls hospitalist Kent to admit Ms. Mann for elevated serum calcium levels.

Kent reviews past records and learns that this elevated calcium level is lower than previous levels. Moreover, the current level is only mildly elevated. Mild elevations in calcium do not lead to kidney damage or other worrisome symptoms. Kent also learns that the woman has primary hyperparathyroidism, a condition characterized by high calcium levels. For mild calcium elevation, the advised treatment is hydration, exercise and limited intake of calcium-rich foods. Kent recommends that Ms. Mann be discharged home from the ED with instructions to maintain adequate hydration and to follow up with her primary physician.

In response, Tom now states that the woman is too weak to walk and, consequently, unable to go home. Surprised by this sudden revelation, Kent agrees to first evaluate her before determining her disposition. Upon his evaluation, Kent finds no neurological or musculoskeletal deficits. Verifying his earlier recommendations for discharge are still best for the woman's care plan, Kent kindly asks her to walk alongside him across the ED. Sixty feet later, unassisted, Ms. Mann easily keeps pace with Kent as they approach Tom.

"So, you can see that she was able to walk all the way here from her bed without any assistance," informs Kent.

"Um, yeah – she can!" agrees Tom.

While Ms. Mann and Kent amble back to her bed, Tom promptly completes discharge instructions.

...

Tom's action suggests that he desired admitting Ms. Mann over all else. The desire to admit sacrificed truth and compromised integrity. ... But why?

It is difficult to think that an experienced practitioner would be freaked by an harmlessly elevated lab result. If the medical evidence did not rattle Tom, then the looming discharge process must have done it.

Discharging patients home is no quick task. The electronic and paper trailing involved consumes anywhere from twenty minutes to an hour (sometimes more if there are numerous medical comorbidities, medications, equipment, providers, and home care / subacute care facilities involved). On the other hand, transferring someone from one intra-hospital department to another is merely a click away. With one click in the EHR, the transferring provider clicks off, freeing himself of further responsibility. All nurses', social workers', as well as the patient's concerns now belong to the clicked-on provider.

One might argue that such a practice frees the emergency physician to field more incoming cases, thus decreasing wait times and improving patient satisfaction ratings. One must then consider the trade-off: how satisfied will that perfectly self-sufficient patient feel about a needless, costly admission that withdrew her from her daily activities (income earning, socializing, family nurturing)? And for what? A click? A self-serving click?

Now consider how Tom's actions showed disregard for his fellow provider, Kent. Tom's actions appear as if he could not care less whether this admission would be a good use of Kent's time and resources. Tom's timely revelation – or, rather, fabrication – suggests that he was banking on a stressed hospitalist's mindless acceptance of some name and a bed number. Kent's diligence disappointed Tom.

Keep in mind, Kent's diligence, like Tom's actions, may have been selfish. Unlike Tom, however, Kent's selfishness favored the best outcome for the patient as well as pacified healthcare's ambitious statistics for excellent patient outcomes. Those highly sought outcomes require appropriate disposition, not some quick click.

hospice is not shorthand for hospitalization

Brought to the emergency room by her family, Ms. Mann, well in her eighties, had been previously diagnosed with severe, end-stage congestive heart failure. During her last hospitalization in another facility, arrangements had been made to discharge her with hospice.

Hospitalist Kent was contacted by ER physician Noah to admit her for dehydration based on the blood tests and questionable pneumonia on chest x-ray. Realizing that Ms. Mann was a hospice patient, Kent did not understand the request for admission.

Kent: You say this patient was recently discharged home on hospice?

Noah: Yes.

Kent: Does the family recognize that admission in this case would go against hospice?

Noah: I don't know. They brought her here, because they want her taken care of.

Kent: But did you ask what their long-term goals are for her condition?

Noah: Look, I've been doing this for a long time. I've been through this rodeo before. These folks brought her in, because they want her to be taken care of. She is dehydrated and has pneumonia and needs to be treated for that!

Kent, who just recently began working at this facility, did not want to ruffle feathers. He relented, recognizing that Noah was not budging. Kent decided to ask the family about their understanding of hospice and their true wishes. Furthermore, Kent suspected the "pneumonia" reported on the chest x-ray was typical fluid accumulation from advanced congestive heart failure. Kent also deduced that the dehydration was expected for a dying patient who stopped eating or drinking. In the latter stages of terminal illnesses, the metabolism diminishes; the body can no longer harvest nutrients. Therefore, the lack of nutrition does not cause suffering.

Kent evaluated Ms. Mann then spoke with the family at the bedside. The family clearly expressed that Ms. Mann's condition "will never get better." Until a few days ago, Ms. Mann was still communicative with the family. She became less communicative over the following days then she stopped speaking altogether. The family confessed they had panicked and brought her to the emergency room without contacting their hospice representative.

Based on Kent's assessment, Ms. Mann, though lethargic, appeared comfortable with no signs of distress on supplemental oxygen. Kent reviewed the natural progression of terminal illness with her family, who listened attentively and, in fact, emphasized hope that Ms. Mann would never suffer throughout this period. They stressed their preference to return her home with hospice care; for, when she had been of sound mind, she declared many times to everyone that she wished to die at home.

Unfortunately, by this time, the hospice organization had closed for the day. Kent had to hospitalize Ms. Mann overnight. The next day, the hospice team reestablished communication with the family to resume hospice care at home. Ms. Mann was discharged later that afternoon to respect her expressed wishes.

■ ■ ■

Presume Noah understood the principles and practices of hospice. So, his motivation to admit Ms. Mann must have been focused on alleviating suffering amid invasive medical treatments, such as needle sticks for IV catheters or labs. Noah must have believed that flooding this dying woman with fluids to completely fill her fluid-dense lungs from end-stage congestive heart failure would help her feel less parched. Then, exposing her to chemicals her failing body could not metabolize effectively to treat a phantom pneumonia would heal her. Noah must have considered all these things when he demanded Ms. Mann be hospitalized. ...There is the possibility that Noah did not fully understand how hospice works; but, given his experience with "this rodeo before," that must not be the case. So, unless Noah was simply an ignorant clinician, it seems he may have simply sought a quick exit from his ER.

What's faster than a discharge muddled with family education / reaffirmation, social workers and hospice facilitators? Yep, an admission. Let Kent sort it out. That is what he is supposed to do – handle all things humane while clinicians handle serum studies and radiographic imaging. After all, Noah should not be bothered with clarifying the family's understanding between hospice and hospitalization. He never asked and had no intentions to ask. "I don't know" was an adequate assessment. He could not bother about the family's long-term goal for Ms. Mann; therefore, he could not deign to answer Kent's questions.

Noah's responses and actions imply assembly line thinking:

> Patient come in.
>
> Next.
>
> Patient get tests.
>
> Next.
>
> Patient get drugs.
>
> Next.
>
> Patient get admitted.
>
> Done.

Why care whether *dying woman get comfort*?

you start it, you finish it – a doc gone rogue

From the ED to the Floor:

Once the Emergency Department determines that a patient requires admission, a text message is sent to the hospitalist triage phone, alerting the admitting physician to call the ED to learn the details about the patient. As soon as the emergency physician relays the information, he immediately relinquishes all patient responsibilities to the receiving hospitalist. So, the sooner the hospitalist personally assesses the patient, the safer the patient will be. The hospitalist is completely liable for a patient he has not yet met.

Emergency physician Ned phoned hospitalist Emmet to admit Mr. Mann. After reviewing the case, Emmet determined that Mr. Mann did not require admission to the hospital. He gave Ned suggestions for treatments prior to discharge home. Annoyed, Ned slammed the phone.

Emmet continued caring for other patients. Roughly one hour later, he received a page from the floor upstairs.

"Hello?"

"We need orders for Mr. Mann who just arrived from the ED," a nurse informed.

Seething, Emmet went to the floor, performed a complete assessment, confirmed his earlier assessment and completed the documentation to discharge a healthy man home.

Emmet reported the incident to his director Monty, who directly emailed Ned about the inappropriateness of his actions:

You sent a patient to another unit without an accepting

physician. That brazen act could have potentially been

devastating for the patient.

Monty included Ned's director Albert in the email thread. Alarmed by the documented events, Albert phoned Monty:

Firmly, Monty explained, "I sent the message to highlight how inappropriate Ned's actions were."

"I completely agree," backed Albert. "In the future, though, just don't put stuff like that in writing. It makes us look bad."

. . .

So, it is perfectly fine to behave badly as long as no one sees the bad behavior. Got it, just like litigation: no documented evidence, no crime to convict.

Now focus on the glaring insult – dismissal of procedure and person if it interferes with one's personal agenda. Whether ED goals, personal vindication, or a need to go home was the reason, Ned roguishly dismissed the point of collaborative healthcare by secretly admitting the patient to the floor.

The sneaky act exposes Ned's intent to force Emmet into compliance with his will despite Mr. Mann's rights. Ned had performed enough handoffs to know that an accepting physician is required prior to transferring a patient. If no one accepts the transfer, the transferring provider (Ned) must continue responsible care. Federal regulations (EMTALA*) are enforced to prevent this dumping. These laws prevent adverse outcomes for severely ill human beings who would be unseen and essentially abandoned.

Without an accepting medical provider for Mr. Mann, the principled course of action requires that *Ned* continue caring for Mr. Mann after *Ned* transferred him out of the ED.

Instead, Ned showed Emmet a thing or two by admitting Mr. Mann under Emmet's name. That darn hospitalist was going to admit someone, because Ned said admit, darn it! Sadly, Emmet faltered beneath Ned's pressure and shuffled priorities to correct Ned's wrongdoing. Perhaps fatigue or fear or ignorance forced Emmet to fold. Despite the reason, Emmet must learn from this so that when he faces another Ned, he will stand his ground and inspire the next Ned to practice responsibly.

*EMTALA – Emergency Medical Treatment and Labor Act

uh, whatever. give 'em antibiotics.

Mr. Mann had persistent hiccups that interfered with his daily functions. The hiccups escalated into intermittent vomiting that burned his chest from recurrent reflux. The burning chest pain caused intense tightening of his throat. He then sought medical help.

In the emergency room, ER physician Ted ordered a cervical CAT scan to rule out a physical obstruction in the neck. No such abnormality was seen. Incidentally, modest irregularities in the partially visualized upper lungs were loosely labeled as, "could be possible pneumonia." Mr. Mann had no fever, cough or any other respiratory symptoms. Still, Ted prescribed Mr. Mann a round of antibiotics.

The following day, Mr. Mann returned to the ER. The hiccups intensified so much so that Mr. Mann vomited after nearly every meal. Repeat labs were unremarkable. Ted worried that the gentleman may develop unstoppable vomiting and, thus, contacted hospitalist Duncan to hospitalize the patient.

Duncan evaluated Mr. Mann and proposed that underlying gastritis (stomach lining inflammation) or an ulcer triggered severe reflux resulting in vomiting. The diaphragm, the large respiratory muscle, which sits above the stomach, must have been irritated in turn. Continual spasms of this muscle resulted in relentless hiccups. Given the persistent vomiting, Duncan reasoned overnight hospitalization with medications to treat the reflux and lessen the hiccups was rational. If those measures failed to improve Mr. Mann's state, endoscopic procedures to search for an ulcer would be the next step. Duncan did not resume antibiotic treatment. He detailed the treatment plan to Mr. Mann and his son.

Curious, Mr. Mann's son clarified, "You're not going to continue his antibiotics?"

To which Duncan replied, "Your father came in with hiccups and got antibiotics. Does that make sense to you?"

Mr. Mann's son chuckled and shook his head.

■ ■ ■

Who knew how certain "could be" and "possible" could be in the absence of any, ANY other clinical signs for active disease? Knee-jerk antibiotic prescribing without conclusive evidence or shrewd suspicion is no longer presumptive medicine but a gamble. Tossing bacterial resistance about like jacks and a rubber ball will ultimately become a game of fatality.

Sometimes, thinking it through is better than an arbitrary prescription for whatever could be possible.

... well, actually, *every* time ...

HOSPITALIST TO NURSE

the note or the order, hmm ...

Twenty-five-year-old Ms. Mann who has developmental delay required hospitalization for aspiration pneumonia due to multiple vomiting episodes. She likely aspirated stomach contents into her lungs during these vomiting spells. Ms. Mann is nonverbal and could not communicate her needs. Hospitalists relied on her physical exam to determine her clinical progress. Given her inability to swallow safely, Ms. Mann required a percutaneous endoscopic gastrostomy (PEG) feeding tube. A PEG tube is inserted through the skin directly into the stomach.

Initially, Ms. Mann's tube feeds were held until the vomiting completely subsided. IV fluids provided hydration during that time. Preemptively, the admitting hospitalist consulted the gastroenterologist for PEG tube adjustments. Fortunately, Ms. Mann's symptoms were due to a stomach virus. Therefore, the gastroenterologist did not need to contribute further input. Her symptoms resolved within 48 hours.

The following day, hospitalist Blake assumed care for Ms. Mann. He determined that she was ready to restart tube feeds. To ensure Ms. Mann would tolerate feedings, Blake ordered to start feeds at a much slower rate than her norm. He intended to reassess her the next day to determine whether the rate could increase to Ms. Mann's home rate.

That next day, Blake, shocked to find that the tube feeds had never been started, pressed nurse Preston for an explanation:

Blake: How come Ms. Mann has not received her tube feeds yet?

Preston: I saw that the note by the gastroenterologist mentioned that he wanted the tube feeds to be held.

Blake: His note was completed on the 15th; and my order was on the 16th. Why was the order disregarded?

Preston: I thought that since he's the specialist, it would be the gastroenterologist who would decide when the feeds could be started.

Blake: And how did you make that determination? Your responsibility is to execute physicians' orders. If you have a question about an order, then ask the doctor who ordered it. You don't disregard the order because of a note you read. A note is not an order! This patient has gone without food for yet another day!

Preston: I'm sorry. I thought he would make the call. I will start her feeds now.

· · ·

There is nothing wrong with thinking; just check before acting. When working within a team, questioning rather than assuming is the best step prior to committing an act or failing to act. The doctor-nurse order-implement practice is globally practiced. Although making executive decisions is instinctive, it is rash to do so in medicine, especially when each person's role is clear. Speculate: who suffers the most when this happens? The hospitalist's ego from being dismissed by the nurse? The nurse's pride after being corrected by the doctor? Or, the person who starves for over 72 hours?

Now, why did Preston follow an outdated note rather than a present-day order? Preston had more confidence in a doctor who had not seen Ms. Mann at all that day over the doctor who did. Why did Preston assume that the gastroenterologist will *make the call*? Preston likely assumed the stomach specialist will dictate the stomach stuff while the hospitalist babysits. Given contemporary practices, that may be a reasonable presumption. Many hospitalists practice auto-click consultation. Such practices have earned Preston's lack of respect. Knee-jerk consulting has given other providers full confidence that the hospitalist needs doctors to manage his patients; the hospitalist is the one to call for admitting, twilight, and discharge orders. Blink-consulting conveys the notion that the hospitalist follows and scribes for the *real* doctors.

Although a number of hospitalists practice consultation medicine, Preston should not have assumed all hospitalists' practice is such. Whether performed or ignored, Preston executed an order – his own. While awaiting the gastroenterologist to make the call, Preston made a call of his own. Unfortunately, that call resulted in another's needless suffering.

OTC symptoms respond to OTC treatments

OTC stands for over-the-counter.

A Simple Headache

On a general hospital ward, a woman treated for an asthma flare develops a headache. The headache does not affect her vision or normal function. Nonetheless, the woman seeks relief and asks her nurse for pain medication. Nurse Tim pages hospitalist Harrison who orders Tylenol.

"Shouldn't we try something stronger?" advises Tim.

"No." Harrison replies.

"So, all you want me to give is Tylenol?"

"Yes. Is Tylenol not appropriate for a headache? If you were at home with a headache, what would you use?"

Another Simple Headache

A young lady admitted for uncontrolled menstrual bleeding due to an underlying genetic bleeding disorder, von Willebrand's disease, complained of headache. The nurse administered Tylenol. When that failed to relieve the headache, the nurse paged the hospitalist, who had not yet evaluated the woman. To the nurse's surprise, the hospitalist ordered ibuprofen, which the nurse dutifully administered. Forty-five minutes later, the hospitalist arrived onto the floor to evaluate the young lady. The nurse reported that neither medication worked and asked to try something stronger.

The hospitalist greeted the young lady then inquired further about her headache.

"Do you drink tea or coffee?"

"Yes, I have my morning coffee every day."

"Have you had coffee since you've been in the hospital?"

"Now that you mention it – No!"

The hospitalist asked that this woman be given a cup of coffee.

"Coffee?" quizzed the skeptical nurse.

An hour after the young woman consumed coffee, the hospitalist returned to assess the status of the headache.

"It's gone!" she triumphantly reported.

The hospitalist entered a formal request for a cup of coffee with all subsequent breakfast trays.

And, Yet Another, Simple Headache

In need of medication for a gentleman's headache, a nurse stopped the hospitalist arriving onto the floor. The hospitalist asked whether the headache was a new occurrence or a chronic condition. If chronic, the hospitalist coached the nurse to ask which medications the person uses at home. The nurse trucked into the gentleman's room while the hospitalist settled within earshot in the dictation room next door. The hospitalist overheard the nurse:

"What do you take for your headaches?"

The man's soft reply was inaudible.

"Oh, okay. How about Norco? Do you take that? I'll see if we can give you that."

Once again, the hospitalist could not hear the reply.

The nurse entered the dictation room stating, "Doctor, he gets headaches like this occasionally at home and takes Tylenol, but this time, Tylenol did not help; can we give him Norco?"

Norco, a habit-forming narcotic, is hardly the class of medication indicated for headaches.

The hospitalist opted for Excedrin, a well-known over-the-counter headache and migraine reliever. A pharmacist sitting next to the hospitalist chuckled in agreement. The hospitalist evaluated the gentleman following treatment with the OTC medication. Not only did the headache completely resolve, it never recurred for the remainder of his hospital stay!

Aching Muscles

Hospitalized then treated with IV antibiotics for cellulitis, a man complains of back discomfort from lying in the hospital bed. In response, nurse Jacob pages hospitalist Mason for medication.

Upon learning the gentleman has no overt pain, Mason asks Jacob what methods have been attempted to adjust the bed. Jacob reports that nothing has been done. Mason suggests providing additional pillows with a heating pad. Jacob insists on pills.

Mason finally recommends to first noninvasively improve the gentleman's comfort and environment, then, if those measures are unsuccessful, try ibuprofen. Jacob responds:

> "Ibuprofen? That's it?!"

A Leg Cramp

A man with kidney failure requiring dialysis to clear excess chemicals and toxins from the body was admitted to the hospital for uncontrolled elevated blood pressure. While receiving treatment for the elevated blood pressure, the gentleman continued his routine dialysis treatments.

One afternoon, the gentleman suddenly complained about a leg cramp to his nurse, Anthony. Anthony paged hospitalist Sean with the concern. Sean quickly reviewed the medical record and noticed that despite kidney failure, the man's electrolytes (potassium, calcium, magnesium, etc.) were balanced. An imbalance of electrolytes can cause muscle cramps or spasms. Sean explained to Anthony that the absence of electrolyte abnormalities suggests a benign, likely random cause that will resolve on its own.

"So, you don't want to give him anything?"

"What do you suppose he needs for a charley horse?"

...

Is the hospital not the place to use everyday solutions for everyday discomforts? For some reason, simple ailments effectively treated with simple measures in one's home now, by just being in a hospital building, require hard-hitting drugs. Tim and Jacob mockingly imply that first-line treatment should not be over-the-counter remedies like Tylenol or ibuprofen. Although both men did not outright demand them, the expectation for narcotics is clear. Their responses spark the question: Why would health-promoting providers push health-depleting narcotics?

To answer this, a better idea about Tim's and Jacob's stances requires delving.

Nurses are key interactions for patients. In the patients' eyes, nurses set the tone for the medical team's behavior and are the most accessible members of the team. Nurses typically have one ear reserved just for their patients. Hence, if their patients clog their ears with continual complaints, nurses will determine a means to quickly pacify their patients. That may include "preemptively" adding aggressive treatments (knocking out a minor ailment with a major agent) to the drug list in anticipation of pain complaints while lessening future disruptions from their other duties.

Addressing pain complaints become trying when caring for a demanding opioid abuser who has learned how to increase his dosages during hospitalization. Such a patient, if indulged, can be aggressive and monopolize one's entire shift. For some nurses, aggressive opioid abusers can cause anxiety and fear, blocking nurses' ability to serve others. Thus, nurses' seeking narcotic solutions makes some sense.

It is no small challenge: one could (A) indulge or overtreat a patient so that one may serve others and complete his ever-growing to-do list versus (B) bear the complaining and resign oneself to accomplishing none of the tasks expected by peers and administrators. The former option turns the nurse into yet another culprit fueling the opioid crisis. The latter compromises the nurse's efficiency and his value as a useful team member or employee. The path nurses choose varies with each nurse's personal experiences with drugs, the prescribing culture during his training, and the prescribing culture of his current work environment.

Both doctors and nurses shape the prescribing culture of their hospital environment through their interdependent actions driven by one fundamental desire – freedom to complete the work that is required. The nurse's decision to indulge or endure the demanding patient often guides the doctor's response to the nurse's page. Although the nurse's decision is primarily influenced by his peers and supervisors, the decision to indulge (quiet) the patient was likely positively reinforced by the burdened physician's, the cursory resident's or the overtaxed intern's decision to indulge (quiet) the nurse. Regardless of its start, the expectation for pill-popping as first-line treatment undermines health caring.

Lastly, not every ill requires a pill. If this notion of "drugs first" is extinguished, then maybe, through cognitive behavioral techniques for a start, human nature can evolve to draw from its own inherent arsenal of healing as first-line treatment.

puckish or precipitative

Cole:

Shortly after hospitalist Cole started his evening shift at 7 PM, he began to admit a 48-year-old gentleman with multiple medical problems. Cole asked the gentleman if he took any medications at home.

"Yes, I gave the list to the nurse."

The hospitalist searched for the medication list, which was nowhere to be found. He asked the gentleman if he could recall the names of any of his medications.

"Nope. There're too many; that's why I keep a list with the names, strengths and instructions on how I should take them. Ask the nurse: I gave him the list."

Cole sighed and wondered, "*Why, why does this habitually happen? And, seriously, where do these dagnab lists run off too?? ... A penny for every single time ... I'd retire!*"

Grayson:

While rounding, hospitalist Grayson answered a page to Nurse A's extension. He was greeted by Nurse B.

"Hi. I was paged to extension 3645."

"That's this number. I'm covering for Nurse A. He's on break. Did you need something?"

"He paged me. Is it regarding a patient?"

"I don't know. He didn't sign out anything to me before he went on break."

"But he just paged me two minutes ago!"

"Oh! I'm sorry. When he comes off break, I will let him know you called."

Grayson hung up, muttering, "*Man! Why so many times ... why do they just run off on break and never sign out to each other first?!*"

Luke:

During his shift, hospitalist Luke paused between admissions to answer a page from Nurse C at 11:11 PM. This was the twelfth page since the start of his shift at 9 PM.

Nurse C asked, "Our patient Mr. Mann is already asleep and was due for his *sleeping* pill at 10 PM. Should I *wake* him up to give it?"

• • •

Hmm, okay. The best explanation for all three accounts could be passive aggression toward hospitalists. The worst possibility would be a cluster of carelessness, flippancy and daftness.

Assuming the former sentiment fueled these interactions, passive aggressive exchanges among coworkers are quite common, if not expected. The push-pull tug-of-war between nurses and doctors is no secret. (It is discussed in secret among both within their respective professions.) The ED nurse could have paid Cole back for any perceived slights from the hospitalist with that missing information. Nurse A may have assumed that like most docs Grayson would take forever to answer his page. Therefore, if Grayson called before Nurse A returned from his break, so be it; it would be fitting if the nurse kept the doc waiting for a change. Nurse C might have figured out that relentless, trivial pages would karmically frustrate Luke. Truly, what better way to exhaust the exhausting than with futility?

On the other hand, if the latter cluster is the reason, a greater concern surfaces:

— Cole's plight —

The greatest gift a patient can gift a medical provider is a detailed list of his or her medications. Those lists are rare, precious gems desired and cherished by treating practitioners. Knowing medication types and doses can reveal toxicity, undertreatment, overtreatment or lack of treatment; this in turn can determine the diagnosis, aid in diagnosing, and guide the treatment plan. Even if someone presented with a completely unrelated medical issue, continuing that person's home regimen is vital to controlling chronic medical conditions. The medical team member not responsible for diagnosis and treatment may not treasure the list; he could easily overlook such valuables that will be replaced by the patient's oral report. Such an assumption discounts the conscientious efforts from patients to ensure correct medical communication; the assumption unreasonably relies on patients' rote memory. With those lists, patients fulfill their contract to provide the most accurate information to support treatment. It is the entire medical team's obligation to respect and match those efforts. Ensuring those lists are directly submitted to the treating team member or accurately entered in the electronic health record (EHR) honors the contract between the patient and the medical team.

— Grayson's challenge —

Now, honoring the contract between medical team members is tricky. Fact: For whichever reason, many doctors are not timely responders to nonurgent matters. Fact: Nurses cannot be expected to halt all duties while awaiting a slow responder. However, the provider (doctor or nurse) seeking another (doctor or nurse) should be expected to have the needed information available when the sought provider answers the call. Respecting everyone's role and duties is a must. Therefore, the *Pager* must be mindful of the *Paged* just as the *Paged* must be mindful of the *Pager*. The *Pager* should either wait until he is available to answer the returned call or equip the person left in his stead with the desired information or question. The *Paged* should return each page as promptly as possible, regardless of the number of incoming pages. After all, pages are necessary evils of the trade.

— Luke's bafflement —

One necessary evil that plagues hospitalized patients is medications scheduled outside usual waking hours. Nurses shoulder the unpleasant task of executing ill-timed medication orders. It is shrewd to check with the physician whether certain medications can be delayed or skipped during these hours. Certain medications, however, need only the shrewdness of the dispenser.

abuse of power

Nurse Connor calls the on-call hospitalist Dean for pain medicine. Connor's patient has been bothering him to increase the dose of his narcotic. Notorious from prior hospitalizations for narcotic requests, the patient's requests typically climax into unruly demands. Aware of this person's history, Dean informs Connor that there is no medical indication to increase the narcotic dose.

Connor sternly replies, "Well, then I'm going to call you every hour."

Appalled, Dean questions, "Is that a threat?!"

Dean remains steadfast and hangs up the phone.

■ ■ ■

Like phone solicitors, Connor is well versed in the art of wear-and-tear persuasion. Connor knows that physicians commonly complain about workflow interruption. He knows that Dean cannot ignore the pager hammering his ear. Aggressive paging would force Dean to eventually comply with whatever Connor requests. The wear-and-tear method is an effective tool transferred from patient to nurse to doctor in this illustration. All three parties seek one end – peace. The patient wants peace from his cravings, the nurse from the patient, and the doctor from the nurse. Dissecting just his tone, Connor's ploy for peace was a "veiled" threat.

Although Connor executes Dean's orders, Connor can passively govern Dean's orders. By exhausting Dean with repeated disruptions, Connor has a great chance of obtaining his peace from the patient. The drawback is the time required to reach the desired end. Connor may have to wait several intervals lasting five or so minutes at a time before paging Dean again and again. Connor discovered a more direct route to reaching his goal by declaring exactly which weapon of persuasion (wear-and-tear) he will use until his demand is met.

Looming intimidations loosely translates into, "I will torture you until you submit." Although this brazen promise is unprofessional, it must be highly successful, because Connor issued his boldly. Despite that consideration, Connor is not the sole wrongdoer in this affair. Physicians who have caved beneath such intimidations are also at fault. Yielding to unacceptable acts positively reinforces the behaviors. Physicians, therefore, further their own torture.

Now, when scrutinizing the entire situation, one sees Connor abusing his duty to inform and communicate with doctors for personal gain (in this case, to mute his riotous, opioid-abusing patient). Had Dean crumpled beneath Connor's intimidations for personal gain, he would have abused his duty to practice proper medicine. Both Connor's and Dean's violations equally undercut their shared obligation – the betterment of the patient.

trigger paging

Urgently, nurse Peter pages hospitalist Bryce about patient Mr. Mann, who complains of chest pain. Bryce mirrors Peter's urgency, asks him to immediately measure the vital signs, and promises a prompt arrival to the bedside. En route, Bryce contemplates the most likely causes – heart attacks, ruptured aneurysms, arrhythmias, blood clots, fluid in the lungs, pneumonia.

Peter has the vital signs but cannot report more information, because, in his rush to alert the physician, he did not investigate further. Bryce shrugs and quickens to the bedside. Bryce asks Mr. Mann to describe his chest pain. Calmly, Mr. Mann describes a heavy pressure that has now completely disappeared.

Once the large bible that had been left atop his chest while sleeping was removed, the pressure improved. Mr. Mann had simply hoped Peter would give him Tylenol for the discomfort.

■ ■ ■

Nurse Peter heard one of a hospital's most troubling pairings: chest and pain. Chest pain due to lethal cardiac or pulmonary sources requires immediate attention. Such emergencies require informed, problem-focused interventions. In those cases, quickening the response time will give anyone suffering grave cardiac or pulmonary distress the best chance for a successful outcome. The incident presented here is not such a case.

Here, those two words triggered a blind reaction by Peter. If Mr. Mann's hope was simply Tylenol, it is unlikely that he asked while distressed. Mr. Mann's capacity to calmly narrate the events leading to his chest pain and desired treatment suggests that a brief conversation alongside the observation of Mr. Mann's unruffled composure could have resulted in an appropriate, timely, and effective treatment response. Instead, this situation expended double the resources (multiple providers completing the task of one) in double the time.

Peter's decision to *just* call the doctor wasted people's time – Mr. Mann's, Peter's own, the hospitalist's, and a dozen of others' (patients and staff who required the hospitalist). Peter did not improve efficiency by failing to assess his patient. Even if busy with several tasks, Peter's duty to fully assess his patient's new medical complaint must become top priority.

Why?

Assessment = *Discerning* Health Care

belongs to the surgeon – hmm, call the surgeon! part 2

Eight-year-old Miss. Mann presented to the hospital after vomiting amid persistent abdominal pain.

In the ER, labs revealed a modestly elevated white blood cell (WBC) count and a significantly elevated C-reactive protein (CRP) level. An elevated WBC count suggests infection. An elevated CRP level suggests inflammation somewhere, anywhere in the body. Miss. Mann's appendix could not be visualized to definitively rule out appendicitis on the ultrasound. This can also occur with normal overlying intestine. Given the elevated lab levels and inconclusive ultrasound, the ED physician contacted the general surgeon, who admitted Miss. Mann under his service overnight for serial abdominal exams.

The surgeon reckoned that if the child had appendicitis, the pain would migrate. In his note, to prevent overstimulation of her gut, he recommended no food or water. He recommended IV fluids and Tylenol then stated he "will check repeat CBC and CRP in the morning."

Pediatric hospitalist Fitzgerald was consulted by the surgeon for management of any medical issues. Fortunately, Miss. Mann was otherwise healthy. Fitzgerald only modified the IV fluid volume and corrected the Tylenol dose based on the child's weight. Fitzgerald concluded Miss. Mann likely had a stomach viurs that would resolve on its own. He seconded overnight monitoring but decided additional tests were unnecessary at that time.

Early the next morning, nurse Bruno called hospitalist Fitzgerald.

Bruno: The surgeon's *note* mentioned CBC and CRP will be
           ordered for the morning. He ordered the CBC but

didn't order the CRP. Do you want to go ahead and order that test?

Fitzgerald: You should contact the surgeon for that order. I did not recommend that test, so I don't intend to order it.

While rounding later that morning, Fitzgerald approached nurse Caleb, who had replaced nurse Bruno.

Caleb: I was told you wanted us to contact the surgeon to order that CRP. I didn't want to wake the surgeon so early in the morning, so I just went ahead and ordered the test anyway.

Fitzgerald: If you ordered any test under my name, I will not sign it, because I did not recommend such a test.

Caleb: But the surgeon put in his *note* that he wanted a test ordered.

Fitzgerald: That's why you should contact the surgeon to order any test that he may have overlooked. I didn't recommend any test based on my assessment. So, I'm not going to simply order one just because it's mentioned in someone else's note. I don't recommend tests that are not necessary. The patient is improving; so, I suggest treating the patient, not the *note*.

Dissatisfied, Caleb walked off.

Fitzgerald shook his head as he reflected on a past confrontation:

Weeks prior when jointly caring for another patient, Caleb had grilled Fitzgerald: "Why are you ordering all these tests? The surgeon had not mentioned any of those tests in his *note*!"

. . .

Hmm ... Two questions spring forth:

First, since when does one from the executing discipline police the notes of the determining discipline, judge the determiner's practice, dismiss the determiner's judgment, and act on his own accord with the assumption that the determiner must comply? In the medical profession, nursing is an executing discipline while doctoring is a determining discipline. The latter is trained to investigate, cogitate and determine orders; the former is trained to observe, report and execute orders.

Second, if a religious man can call on his god any hour of the day, why can a nurse not call on his on-call surgeon any hour of the shift?

inconvenient boundaries

Twenty-nine-year-old Mr. Mann presented with sickle cell crisis. Desperately in need of intravenous hydration, a routine peripheral IV catheter had been inserted in his arm. Somehow, the catheter dislodged. Several attempts to reestablish peripheral venous access failed. Hospitalist Ferris consulted pulmonary/critical care intensivist Denton to establish central venous access into a larger, deeper vein. Denton successfully inserted a central line.

Mr. Mann improved slowly, but before he turned the corner, he accidentally pulled the central line. His crisis worsened. Attempts to access his veins peripherally failed, again. Hospitalist Ferris could not reach intensivist Denton who had left for the day. Ferris considered solutions: he could ask Denton to return to the hospital or ask the ED physician to insert a new central line.

Meanwhile, the nurses told their supervisor Gary. Within minutes, Gary asked competitor intensivist David to insert the line. During David's procedure Denton entered the room. Angered by the site of the competitor, Denton was exasperated. Neither Gary nor David had talked to Denton. Once he learned the matter, hospitalist Ferris was incensed by David's encroachment and Gary's rashness.

■ ■ ■

Five tiers of trespasses exist here: Nurse to Hospitalist, Nurse Supervisor to Hospitalist, Subspecialist to Nurse Supervisor, Subspecialist to Hospitalist, Subspecialist to Subspecialist.

Tier 1 – Nurse to Hospitalist

The first communication breakdown occurred between the nurses and hospitalist Ferris. Before appealing to the nurse supervisor, the nurses needed to ask Ferris whether he had a plan in play. If Ferris had no plan, the nurses should have informed him that they needed to report this to their supervisor given the urgent need for IV access. Then again, what if the nurses' attempts to speak with Ferris failed for whatever reason (a fatal emergency called overhead, discussions with other specialists to resolve the matter, or outright snubbing)? The nurses must alert those who will address the matter. Reporting the event to their supervisor is expected ... provided it is objective, factual reporting.

Tier 2 – Nurse Supervisor to Hospitalist

If Gary felt so inclined to intervene for his nurses, he should have collaborated with Ferris. Instead, Gary chose an uncommunicative method that heightened the discord between competing subspecialists, Denton and David. Rather than create a cooperative culture among providers, Gary ignited a hostile one.

Tier 3 – Subspecialist to Nurse Supervisor

As soon as intensivist David spoke with supervisor Gary, he needed to immediately redirect Gary to hospitalist Ferris before entertaining the discussion. This requires David be fair and just in his practices, particularly in the acquisition of patients.

Tier 4 – Subspecialist to Hospitalist

After redirecting nurse supervisor Gary to hospitalist Ferris, intensivist David could have either waited until he heard from hospitalist Ferris or contacted him directly.

Tier 5 – Subspecialist to Subspecialist

Intensivist David could have courteously notified fellow intensivist Denton about the nurse supervisor's call. Again, this suggestion requires David's practice be just and fair.

Still, if only one tier governs this battery of offenses, it would be the lack of communication from the nurse supervisor.

Focus solely on the urgency for intravenous access: the quicker one acts, the sooner the resolution. For convenience, nurse supervisor Gary tagged the nearest white coat to resolve the matter. Gary's primary objective may have been to prevent worsening of Mr. Mann's crisis. He may have prioritized patient care over all else. Gary's motives could have been sincere duty and compassion. It is possible, however, that Gary might have succumbed to egoism or self-inflation. Who knows how weary Gary may have been from constantly righting the slipups of all those bungling hospitalists throughout that entire week? No longer able to suffer through yet another useless exchange, Gary may have decided to bypass that blundering lot and get that much needed central line. In no time, Gary saved his panicked nurses, the suffering patient, the maladroit doctor and the day overall. Whichever the motive, Gary failed to anticipate the repercussions of reacting shortsightedly.

Wait – how much time was saved between Denton's arrival and the completion of David's procedure? Hmm, David had not completed the procedure prior to Denton's arrival. Fifteen to twenty minutes likely lapsed. So, fifteen to twenty minutes of patience following shrewd collaboration would have prevented the insults inflicted upon all involved. One can only wonder what that next day at work must have been like …

agenda before consideration

Hospitalist Ross cringed beneath the overhead announcement – CODE WHITE!

A child was dying. In seconds, a nurse paged him that a 7-year-old found unresponsive in the field was headed their way. Simultaneously, the ED called echoing the same.

Ross burst into the ED just as the unresponsive little girl was wheeled to a private area. The emergency physician posted himself at the head of the bed to secure the child's airway. Ross ran the code, delegating resuscitation actions among the other medical teammates. The interosseous catheter placed on the right tibia failed to administer medications. Instead, immediate subdermal swelling occurred as fluid infiltrated the skin. Ross noticed bruising on that right tibia and presumed it was EMT's attempts to place a catheter. Instantly, a new catheter site was secured on the left tibia through which medications were administered.

After three minutes of resuscitation, Ross asked the whereabouts of the mother. She was en route to the hospital. Ross left the emergency physician in charge of the code to speak with the mother once she arrived. Soberly, he gently explained the bleak outlook despite their efforts. The stunned mother just stared at Ross. Understanding that she may need the closure other families have received by being present as medical providers fight to bring their family member back, Ross invited her into the room. Ross resumed the lead and concentrated on the child. The mother had only glanced at her child before someone shooed her out of the room.

Fifteen minutes passed before the sense of loss descended upon the team. Ross again asked the emergency physician to take the lead. He searched for the mother to review the events and the team's intent to settle the code. Just as Ross parted his lips, nursing supervisor Mack swooped in.

"Uh, excuse me. Uh – that bruise on her leg – did she come in with that – did she have that bruise at home – when did she get that bruise on her leg?"

Aghast, Ross glared at Mack speechlessly. He could not believe Mack's interrogating this stunned mother who needed to first absorb that her child did not survive after thirty-five minutes of CPR then process that her child was dead. Ross knew that the bruise required further investigation. He chose to focus on the mother's acceptance of the death of her child. Ushering her away from Mack, Ross offered to escort her back into the room. The mother nodded, wishing to say goodbye to her daughter. They entered right as the code was called to an end.

Some other person yelled out, "You can't be in here!" That person rushed her out of the room. Several minutes later, the emergency physician, social worker and Ross settled down with the mother in a quiet, private place to discuss the events leading to her unresponsive child.

■ ■ ■

Mack's insensitivity toward a bewildered, newly grieving parent does not need to be stressed here.

Instead, the disconnection among the medical team during an emotional trauma requires scrutiny. Take the revolving door, for instance. Permitting the mother to enter then yelling at her to leave then readmitting the mom into the room then rushing her out agitated a highly sensitive situation. The warring messages expose a disjointed medical team. Often different medical disciplines draw from different schools of thought on ethical matters. Whether a parent will benefit or worsen after witnessing his child's resuscitation can never be determined unanimously. Every person hones coping skills unique to himself. Measures that serve one person well may be unhealthy for another.

Ross' experience with resuscitation and associated grief prompted him to ask the mother if she wished to witness the events then say her goodbyes. Whoever charged her out of the room both times may have had different experiences. No right or wrong exists in the decision to permit or omit a parent's viewing the resuscitation of her child. However, denying her wish to be with her dying child favors wrong over right. Strangers do not know what will help her process the loss. Heck, the parent, herself, may not know if seeing everything will help her. Still, it is her loss and, therefore, her call.

Given the revolving sequence, mother in then mother out, there must not have been a formal hospital policy to follow. So, in the absence of an established directive, how could this team have prevented that confusion? The burden falls upon the leader. Although most individuals are natural leaders, the one responsible for the resuscitation (or running the code) is the leader who must make this call. As the code leader delegates duties, he must manage the attendance and the tempo of the room. Ross needed to inform everyone to make room for the mother. A brief announcement about the mother's authorization to remain in the room could have prevented contradictions in patient-provider communication.

Another error in patient-provider communications occurred the moment Mack interrupted his colleague relaying delicate information to play hardnosed detective. Besides undermining his fellow provider's authority and time, Mack's tactless interference likely initiated distrust between the medical team and the patient's mother, as well as worsened provider-provider relations. No one, no matter the setting, takes kindly to curt interruptions. Mack needed a suitable moment to strike during his ruthless pursuit of the truth for justice or documentation. If Mack insisted on charting an exposé, he should have followed the emergency physician, social worker and Ross' lead - find the right place at the right time as a team.

a bird's eye

The Process:

Admitting a patient from the ED can take a hospitalist thirty minutes to two hours (or longer) depending on the complexity of the admission. The simplest admission to the intensive care unit (ICU) takes at least one hour to complete. In this hospital, once the hospitalist determines whether the patient's condition requires hospitalization, the ED physician requests a bed on "the floor." The hospitalist completes his assessment; orders tests and medications; then finalizes the admission. The patient is shuttled from the ED to the floor, freeing an ED bed for new patients. Oftentimes, pending admissions fill the queue and nurses on the floor may need the hospitalist to address pressing issues before he has an opportunity to assesses the patient. The hospitalist must juggle the various camps by providing general instructions to manage floor patients awaiting a formal admission while completing each admission as efficiently as possible.

The Night Shift:

When hospitalist Miles began his night shift, hospitalist Victor, who was finishing his evening shift, said he still had three patients to see and would be unable to tackle two new pending admissions. Miles buckled down, ready to dive into both of Victor's hand-offs. Just before he could log the first initial, the ED messaged that three ED physicians needed to endorse more admissions. The first doctor rattled off three new admissions, the second detailed two others, and the third tacked on one more. Three from this new crop of admissions required critical care management in the ICU. So, within a span of twenty minutes, Miles' night exploded into *eight* pending admissions! Miles' best-case scenario would be to complete these *8* admissions – three of which were for critically ill patients – in *7* hours as he fielded the expected flood of overnight cross-coverage calls for established patients.

Miles choked back his panic as he embarked upon his feat. He desperately hoped the ED did not call with more admissions. He then prayed that none of the floor patients would suddenly crash. By midnight, three hours deep into his shift, Miles miraculously started his fourth admission. A curious page from nurse supervisor Don demanded his prompt reply.

> Don: Hi Dr. Miles, I was wondering when you will get to see patient Mann.
>
> Miles: He's on my list of many; I haven't gotten to him yet.
>
> Don: Well, can you get to him as soon as possible? He's been waiting a long time.
>
> Miles: Uh, is there something that needs to be addressed right now?
>
> Don: No; I just noticed that he was sent up from the ED hours ago, and you still haven't seen him yet.
>
> Miles: I'm working as fast as I can. Unless there is a life-threatening emergency, please do not ever call me with such a request ever again!

Hours passed. Miles sprinted from admission to admission. Bits of fare were wedged within charting orders. Only five minutes had been spared for bladder relief the entire night. By seven in the morning, ten hours later, Miles wondrously tucked in *10* new floor patients and rescheduled one patient's final date with destiny during a code. Whew!

■ ■ ■

Yay for Miles, the tragic hero, for triumphing over such an exploit.

But … my, my, he was a bit snippy about it. After all, Don simply asked when Miles would see a patient who needed to be seen. Consider Don's point: As the nurse supervisor, he must coordinate the workflow among the nurses while ensuring proper hospital floor assignment for patients coming from the ED. To foster a steady, productive workflow, Don must resolve any barriers to transitioning then settling new patients to the floors. He therefore must identify the root hindering this goal. Often, that root culprit is the admitting physician. Undoubtedly, Miles' delay in placing orders hindered the rest of the medical team's productivity as well as patient Mann's ability to acclimate to his new environment. From Don's view, it might have been difficult to figure out Miles' priorities.

But … surely, surely, Don knew Miles – the legally liable teammate - was equally, if not more, aware that a patient (and several more beyond Don's care) required apt assessments and orders. If Don had considered this fact and desired to just plant a bug in Miles' ear to gingerly nudge him, would it have been *absolutely* necessary to interrupt Miles with the obvious? Perhaps Don was advocating for patient Mann. Perhaps Don was frustrated with his staff's stagnation. Perhaps Don questioned Miles' priorities and ethics. Perhaps, in response to all these musings, Don lessened his frustrations with a pinch of passive aggression disguised as an innocent question.

Clearly both individuals were pressed by a common stressor – settling newly admitted patients to the floors. Before their shifts' end, both parties must clear their interdependent "to-settle" list. Don's apprehension is understandable. His approach, however, could have been tweaked a bit.

If Don desperately required reassurance that Miles prioritized his patient (or check box), he could have phrased his question collaboratively:

> "Hi Dr. Miles, I have patient Mann up here. It looks as if he's been
> here for a couple of hours. How are things looking for you? Is there
> a window of time I can help prepare the patient for your arrival?"

Instead, he issued a command in the tone of an overseer directing his charge to action.

Despite the dismay at a command from an unauthorized figure, Miles, too, could have versed his perspective and requirements collegially:

> "As soon as possible. Unfortunately, there are several others in patient Mann's position. It's just been so busy today, as I'm sure you well know. But, hey, I have him on my radar; and if all goes well with those before him, I can get to him in good time. To get to it, I need to stay off this phone. Please let me know of any near-death events I need to stop and take a call for. Otherwise, the next time we speak, I'll be able to tell you Mr. Mann is good to go."

Now, that approach may not prevent another phone call, but the message is clear, informative and kind (enough).

Both providers need to remember that they are dealing with the same stressors from different angles. If one of the two could have homed in on their common ground and redirected the conversation to a supportive, collaborative discussion, a mutually satisfying conclusion may have been achieved.

paging Dr. X, paging Dr. X

- Doctor ordered a CT with contrast.

  > Nurse: Doctor, who will consent for the patient to have this
  > CT?
  >
  > Doc: The patient will.

- The patient wanted to leave AMA (Against Medical Advice).

  > Nurse: Yes, but his wife does not want to take him home, so
  > ...?
  >
  > Doc: That's between the wife and the patient.

- The patient locked himself in the bathroom.

  > Nurse: He refuses to come out.
  >
  > Doctor: What do you want me to do?
  >
  > Silence
  >
  > Doc: Call security!

- The patient had orders for a regular diet.

  > Nurse: Is it okay to give the patient ice chips?

- A lab test returned slightly abnormal at 7:30 AM. The day, rounding hospitalist works from 7 AM to 7 PM. He thought the slight abnormality was inconsequential and required no action. In the middle of the following night at 2 AM:

  > Nurse: The bicarb from earlier is a little low.
  >
  > Doc: When was that lab drawn?
  >
  > Nurse: At 7:30 AM.

Doc: Did the daytime doc, who handled these daytime labs, say anything?

Nurse: I don't know.

Doc: Did you check the notes and orders?

Nurse: No.

- The following orders were placed: "discontinue IV when tolerating orals and urine is clear."

Nurse: Should I discontinue the IV fluid?

Doc: Is she eating well?

Nurse: Yes.

Doc: Is the urine clear?

Nurse: Yes.

- Night nurse peruses the patient's chart. Two days ago, the magnesium level was low. The nurse pages the cross-cover hospitalist at 3 AM.

Nurse: Will any replacements be done for that magnesium, Doctor?

Doc: From two days ago??

- The patient was observed in his private room.

Nurse: Doctor, the patient is masturbating.

- At 5 AM, the patient wanted to leave AMA. The nurse instantly pages the cross-cover hospitalist.

Nurse: He wants to leave at 8 AM when his mother will be able to take him home.

Doc: Oh, so well after seven, when the rounding hospitalist, who takes care of him will be here?

- A magnesium protocol had been implemented to instruct staff in correcting abnormal levels. The hospitalist ordered the protocol in conjunction with a magnesium serum level. The test returned low at 0.9.

  Nurse: The magnesium level is 0.9.

  Doc: What does the protocol say?

  Nurse: To give 4 grams IV of magnesium if the level is less than 1.1.

  Doc: Did you give it?

  Nurse: No.

  Doc: Why not?

  Silence.

- The nurse text pages the hospitalist:

  Re 308B – Can CT be ordered/done without contrast? Pt is hard stick, attempted CT with contrast did not go well.

  ... but ... The contrast needed to rule out pulmonary embolism.

- The patient had a complaint. The nurse notified the hospitalist.

  Nurse: The patient complained of abdominal pain yesterday but doesn't have any complaints today.

  Silence.

- The hospitalist admitted a patient for diarrhea with orders to test the stool. Within the hour, the nurse paged the hospitalist.

  Nurse: The patient is having diarrhea.

  Doc: That's what I'm admitting the patient for.

  Nurse: Yes, I know. I just wanted you to know the patient still has diarrhea.

- The patient started hemodialysis. The nurse paged the hospitalist.

  Nurse: The patient has not peed.

  Doc: That's why he's on dialysis.

- The patient on BiPAP (a special breathing device) could not catch his breath. The nurse urgently paged the hospitalist. The hospitalist charged to the bedside. The BiPAP mask had not been secured and tightened onto the patient's face. The hospitalist tightened the mask.

  Doc: How's that? Is the breathing better?

  Patient: Yes.

- Nurse approaches the hospitalist to answer another question from the patient in room 14.

  Doc: What question does he have?

  Nurse: I didn't ask him.

  Annoyed by so little effort and information, the hospitalist addressed the urgent medical matter himself.

  Doc: Your nurse said that you had a question for me.

  Patient: Yes! I was wondering if I could get one of those yellow socks?

- The hospitalist was meeting with the team in the conference room for collaborative rounds. Another nurse, out of turn, interrupted the group in a fright.

  Nurse: The patient was pronounced dead earlier. Yeah, but I don't think he's dead!

  The hospitalist leapt to his feet and raced to the bedside.

  The patient was lying ...

  in a body bag ...

zipped up.

The hospitalist unzipped the body bag.

Doc: Yep, still dead.

HOSPITALIST TO ADMINISTRATION

psst, protocols don't think; pass it on

Case 1:

A 65-year-old woman enduring metastatic colon cancer required emergency treatment with potent IV steroid dexamethasone to acutely decrease brain swelling.

Within days of her hospitalization, she developed shortness of breath. Her underlying malignancy increased her risk for pulmonary embolism (lung blood clots). In response, the hospitalist ordered an urgent contrast-enhanced CAT scan. The radiology technician rejected this order quoting the hospital protocol's requirement for "prepping" patients with the steroid prednisone to prevent an adverse reaction to the contrast. Per protocol, the prednisone must be administered 13 hours prior to the scan then again one hour before.

The hospitalist phoned the technician:

Hospitalist: The patient has actually been on another steroid, dexamethasone, for the past four days, so she's essentially "prepped" for the CAT scan.

Technician: Our protocol requires that she receive prednisone first. So, she can't get the CAT scan yet.

Hospitalist: I understand; but the dexamethasone is, in fact, eight times stronger than prednisone, so she'll be fine.

Technician: Yeah, well, I can't let her get the test because our protocol requires prednisone.

Frustrated, the hospitalist asked to speak with the radiologist. Upon speaking with the hospitalist, the radiologist readily agreed the woman was more than ready to safely complete the CAT scan with contrast.

Case 2:

A man hospitalized for a massive pulmonary embolism was immediately treated with a blood thinning heparin infusion. Additional testing discovered an abdominal tumor requiring biopsy to determine its type and treatment. The interventional radiology staff quoted their protocol requirement to stop blood thinners (anticoagulants) for a minimum of 24 hours prior to any biopsy procedure.

Different classes of anticoagulants have different elimination rates. Knowing heparin's four-hour elimination rate once stopped, the hospitalist was assured his patient could complete the procedure safely without prolonged interruption of the anticoagulant. The interventional radiology administrator, a physician, agreed that the protocol delayed care and posed potential danger in this patient. The administrator directly approved the initiation of the procedure four hours following the interruption of heparin.

■ ■ ■

Like a map of the wilderness, protocols are helpful guides. And, just like that map, protocols can assist in navigating typical scenarios from which guidelines are drafted. In the wild, what happens when the landscape is drastically altered due to inclement weather? In that case, that map is spectacularly useless. And, just like that map, protocols serve as inadequate guides when treating exceptional individuals.

Although both scenarios occur in the radiology suite, the myth of an *absolute protocol* is practiced in all departments. The debunking of an absolute protocol requires a power superior to some measly doc; it demands the omnipotent – Administration! Administrators are those neutral directors whose sights lie beyond the protocol and the patient. With such a grand scope, administrators can appreciate the varying degrees of medical knowledge among all practitioners. They can draft protocols that allow the system and its substrates to operate without minute-to-minute direction. Most protocol-driven systems can independently function for extended periods, but they do require periodic review, revision and education.

For instance, the two preceding cases could have resulted in morbidity or mortality if the myth of absolute protocol had been followed. During review of poor outcomes, how often will Administration consider the protocol as a possible culprit? If the protocol is the problem, will time and resources be allocated for revisions? Or, if the protocol is enforced as an absolute law, how will administrators prevent human error in exceptional cases?

Given their grasp of medical knowledge disparities among their staff, administrators have an advantage over staff. While physicians and technicians operate from their respective positions, administrators can weigh both perspectives to improve future outcomes. Administrators can underscore in written protocols that physicians, physician assistants and nurse practitioners may override a protocol as their education, training and experience determine. They can then periodically stress this point during staff meetings. When a protocol enforcer questions the clinician, that individual could be instructed to first contact his supervisor or directly connect the clinician with the administrator before a flat refusal. Educating staff about two principles will empower the protocol enforcers and the protocol itself:

(1) Absolutes cannot anticipate every loophole
(2) Exceptions to the protocols *indeed* exist.

collaborative rounds: the rounds that just keep rounding

Collaborative Rounds:

The assigned nurse, the assigned case manager/social worker, the charge nurse, a pharmacist (often with a student in tow), a physical therapist, and the assigned hospitalist comprise the collaborative medical rounding team. Rounds occur at the bedside, permitting all members, as well as the patient, to contribute and proceed in one accord toward the patient's care goals and plan.

7:00 AM – Pre-rounds

Hospitalist Forrest juggled the droves of floor pages ranging from urgent to routine while sorting through the histories, progress notes, test results, and overnight events of the patients he had been assigned.

9:00 AM – Physician Rounds

Forrest hustled to personally interview, examine and update his sixteen patients while sorting through numerous floor pages ranging from urgent to routine.

10:00 AM – Collaborative Rounds

The medical team entered the first patient's room. Charge nurse Herbert introduced the entire team by title and name. Patient Mr. A Mann in room 404 quickly awakened to receive all seven people hovering over him. Herbert continued to explain the visit as an opportunity to learn the general plan and instructed Mr. Mann to ask questions freely. Assigned nurse Brooks briefed the room with Mr. A Mann's admission events, relevant medical history, care summary and overnight course. Forrest then outlined the working diagnosis, his treatment plan, the pending tests and his likely discharge in two days. Mr. A Mann in 404 asked questions, which the team answered before exiting. Immediately in the hall, case manager Gerald asked when Mr. A Mann will be discharged.

Forrest faced Gerald and repeated, "Just like I said, in two days."

To which Gerald replied, "Oh, okay."

Once charge nurse Herbert entered the hall, he stopped Forrest and inquired, "Is the patient going to be here another day, doc?

Forrest faced Herbert and repeated, "Just like I said, in two days."

The team proceeded. Brooks summarized the events leading to the admission of Mr. B Mann in 408.

"...The patient came in with pneumonia – "

"No. Mr. B Mann is here, because he has a blood clot in his lung." Forrest corrected.

Brooks continued to rattle off overnight events, test results and scheduled procedures.

After the team finished their briefing in turn, Mr. Mann was invited to ask questions.

"So, what about my pneumonia?"

"You do not have pneumonia," Forrest clarified. "There is a blood clot in your lungs."

"Then why did the nurse say I have pneumonia?"

"The ER thought you had pneumonia, but now, your latest tests did not show pneumonia. We now know for sure that you don't have pneumonia; but what you do have is a blood clot in your lungs that we are treating with medicines to control that clot," Forrest clarified.

"Oh, okay. I see."

Forrest concluded the visit, "You are doing much better. Anticipate we will discharge you tomorrow. What other questions do you have?"

"None."

As the team exited the room, Gerald asked Forrest, "So, is the patient going home today, Doctor?"

"No, just like I said, the patient will be here till tomorrow. The patient will go home tomorrow."

The team proceeded onto the third room. After conducting the standard briefing, case manager Gerald announced before everyone that the patient is not safe to go home.

"So, we are working on getting a place for him to go to," Gerald finished.

Forrest turned to Mr. C Mann in 411, "They are going to get back to you with options for which facilities you may want to go to for short-term rehab. Medically, you are okay to go home today, but we will need to keep you until we find a place for you. Sometimes it can be done in a few hours or in a few days."

"So," Brooks questioned, "can this patient go home today?"

Forrest turned his attention from Mr. C Mann to Brooks, "No, we just talked about the fact that the patient can't go home but is going for rehab."

The team proceeded from room to room, switching nurses based on patient assignments until all sixteen patients had been seen. At the conclusion of rounds, the team peeled away leaving the physician, charge nurse and case manager in conference. Forrest summarized the rounds:

"Discharge patients in room 3, 7, and 10. Room 11 needs a PT eval to determine short-term rehab. Room 12 needs a referral for a homeless shelter …" Forrest rattled off floor transfers, telemetry requirements and the like. After, everyone scattered off to his respective tasks.

11:00 AM – Documentation

Forrest started on his progress notes. Within an hour, a few floor pages interrupted him with questions about transfers and dispositions that had been addressed during collaborative rounds then summarized during the huddle.

The Next Day

Forrest conducted his day just as the day before in preparation for collaborative rounds.

10:00 AM – Collaborative Rounds

The team reached room 408 housing Mr. B Mann treated for a pulmonary embolism. Brooks again launched into his spiel.

"...The patient came in with pneumonia – "

"No. Remember yesterday when we went through this? Mr. Mann has blood clots – " Forrest corrected.

"What?! It seems no one knows what I have. Some say I have pneumonia; some say I have blood clots. I feel like nobody knows what they're doing!" punctuated Mr. B Mann.

Derailed, Forrest immediately leapt into damage control. He spent an extra ten minutes explaining how many conditions often present the same way leading to one diagnosis until in-depth testing either confirms the initial diagnosis or reveals another.

"So, yes, Mr. B Mann, when you first came in with shortness of breath, pneumonia seemed likely. But after more tests, the CAT scan revealed you have a blood clot in your lungs and did not show any findings of pneumonia. So, now we know you don't have pneumonia."

Incensed, Mr. B Mann fired, "Well, I don't understand why the nurse keeps saying I have pneumonia when I don't."

Nurse Brooks stood back quietly, neither taking nor correcting the notes he had recited.

After quite some time the team settled the discord with Mr. B Mann in 408. During that time charge nurse Herbert idly witnessed the events. Forrest asked Herbert which of his nurses and assigned patients is up next. Having failed to organize his staff, Herbert left the team waiting for over fifteen minutes as he guessed and searched for the next nurse. One was off the floor, another in the bathroom, a third emerged from the ice vending room.

"Hey," Herbert called out, "are you ready for rounds?"

Forrest addressed the nurse on Herbert's behalf, "Let's round." He faced Herbert and reminded him, "We all know we should be ready to be called from 10-11 to round." Forrest returned to the next nurse, "You're next for rounds. Let's go."

11:45 AM - Documentation

As Forrest reviewed the chart for Mr. B Mann in 408, he saw no diagnosis of pneumonia … *anywhere*.

"What? So, where did Brooks get pneumonia from?"

Minutes after, a case manager named Felix cornered Forrest.

"Do you mind if we run the list, Doctor?"

"Well, actually, I ran the list with your colleague, Gerald, yesterday. Do you not want me to run the list with him?"

"Well, actually, he might call you to run the list as well, but I just figured I'd run the list with you, too."

Forrest sighed, "I'm going to run this list one time with one person since you both work together. So, which one do you want it to be? Do you want it to be with you or with Gerald? Because, if I run the list twice with everybody, I'll never get to the patients."

■ ■ ■

Collaborative rounds assemble the different disciplines that form the patient's care network for clear and coordinated treatment.

It seems to grant everyone access to the treatment and post-hospital plans, while giving everyone an opportunity to participate. It also seems to require nothing of its participants other than to be physically present. Participants need not contribute (or listen for that matter). The questions that spilled tandemly within a breath's span regarding the discharge of Mr. Mann in 404 illustrates such. This was again illustrated in Room 408 and again in Room 411.

Collaborative rounds assemble the different disciplines that form the patient's care network for timely execution of treatment and safe discharge.

Meeting as a group should eliminate redundancy, because the entire plan for the entire patient census is openly discussed at once. If so, why did Forrest receive interruption upon interruption during his documentation time with questions that had already been "discussed"? Also, every department is present for collaborative rounds; thus, every department has a liaison responsible to relay information to the others in his department. Liaisons are typically one person appointed to timely disseminate information to the rest of his colleagues. Why, then, did case manager Felix hamper Forrest's progression of treatments and discharges to review all the patients that should have been reviewed with his fellow case manager Gerald? Perhaps, collaboration is a ruse to "keep those docs in line."

Collaborative rounds assemble the different disciplines that form the patient's care network to reduce confusion and errors.

Brooks must have missed that bit. Not only did he manage to present erroneous information, he managed to regurgitate that error the next day. Brooks failed to communicate accurate information. The treatments and orders could have confused him. To correct his understanding, Brooks simply needed to listen during rounds then scratch *pneumonia* off his scrap of paper and replace it with *blood clot*. Then again, it is up to the physician after all. Brooks just executes the orders. The doc is supposed to know what's what, as he is the liable one anyway. Collaborative rounds that cannot prevent propagation of erroneous information are just befuddling get-togethers.

Collaborative rounds assemble the different disciplines that form the patient's care network to improve patient communication and satisfaction.

Given the upset Brooks' misinformation created, it seems collaborative rounds impaired patient communication and heightened distrust. Truly, how could Mr. B Mann have confidence in his "care" team who appeared to not have cared to be accurate *and* be consistent *and* be on the same page?

So, are collaborative rounds, which assemble the different disciplines that form the patient's care network, designed to (1) further immediate redundancy at bedside, (2) promote delayed redundancy throughout the remainder of the workday, (3) accelerate confusion through the propagation of errors, as well as (4) dissolve patients' confidence and trust in the medical team?

Hmm, sort of seems as such somehow ...

ticked box discharge

Mr. Mann had been hospitalized when he developed extreme delirium and agitation from severe alcohol withdrawal. His harmful impulses required an enclosure bed for his own safety. An enclosure bed is a zipped canopy bed. It prevents climbing out of bed, falls and other injuries.

Prior to hospitalization, Mr. Mann stored a lighter in his shoe. Amid his delirium, he woke to find himself trapped. Instinctively, Mr. Mann seized the lighter, razed his cage and escaped. Fire alarms blared throughout the building. Staff charged to the room, finding flames scaling the canopy toward the ceiling.

The authorities instantly contained the fire before anyone was harmed. Administrative director Chuck declared this man a danger to himself and everyone else. Chuck decided he belonged in a psychiatric facility. Assigned hospitalist Heathcliff stressed that Mr. Mann was too medically volatile to transfer to a dedicated psychiatric unit with untreated, acute alcohol withdrawal. Heathcliff insisted Mr. Mann needed high doses of benzodiazepines and may even require transfer to the ICU (intensive care unit) for continuous IV administration of benzodiazepines. Heathcliff denied discharge. Instead, he consulted the intensivist who agreed that Mr. Mann needed continuous IV benzodiazepines.

Finished for the day, Heathcliff retired home. A page from the hospital interrupted his dinner. He was instructed to finalize Mr. Mann's discharge paperwork so that transportation to the psychiatric hospital could be arranged. Minutes later, the staff paged "never mind now." Administrator Chuck had arranged transportation. Stunned, Heathcliff did not understand this rushed medical discharge override. Discharges to another facility require a comprehensive discharge summary and completion of specific forms. Heathcliff did not perform any of those steps. Somehow, Chuck contrived Mr. Mann's removal.

An hour later, Heathcliff answered a call from the county psychiatric hospital complaining about the transfer of a medically unstable patient with acute alcohol withdrawal in dire need of detoxification treatments. Having not discharged Mr. Mann in the first place, Heathcliff readily agreed to have him returned and admitted to the ICU for continuous IV treatment.

Four days later, Mr. Mann bared semblances of his sober self.

■ ■ ■

Disruption identified. Disruption removed. Box ticked.

Chuck's management appeared so black-and-white. He made medical moves without medical judgement. Perhaps he panicked. Really, what did Heathcliff know? Had the matter been left to the medically trained professional, the hospital would not have been rid of the dangerous arsonist … for the few hours he had been gone.

Perhaps, conversely, the intent to remove a problem long enough to prevent further disruptions … for those few hours … motivated Chuck's medical recklessness.

Bottom line, Chuck was Administration. Administration has the final say. Whether medically sound or medically futile, Administration's box *will* be ticked.

policy emasculates medicine

Case 1:

Due to longwinded tobacco use, Mr. Mann developed chronic obstructive pulmonary disease (COPD) that exacerbated during winter months. Admitted for such an exacerbation, Mr. Mann required oxygen and bronchodilator treatments to help him breathe.

Hospitalist Nate entered Mr. Mann's room, but Mr. Mann was nowhere in sight. The nurse cavalierly reported that Mr. Mann had gone out to smoke and could be seen at the facility's smoking booth outside. Nate, recently employed at this facility, was confused. He could not reconcile how someone admitted for breathing complications from smoking was permitted to smoke. Nate asked the nursing supervisor about it and was educated that the hospital could not infringe upon individuals' rights to smoke if so desired.

Case 2:

Rampant diabetes and dwindling kidney function ushered Ms. Mann into the hospital. She was dangerously short of breath as fluid filled her lungs. Her blood revealed abnormal electrolyte levels. Her sky-high blood sugars worsened her electrolyte abnormalities. Her potassium soared; her bicarbonate dropped, threatening cardiac arrest if not reversed. Meanwhile, the fluid welling in her lungs threatened to intrinsically "drown" her.

Ms. Mann needed dialysis. No, Ms. Mann needed multiple rounds of dialysis. She also needed nonstop, intravenous insulin infusions to whip those blood sugars into a safer range. Her uncontrolled diabetes and renal dysfunction required a specific diet to control her carbohydrate, potassium and magnesium intake.

Paying *those* doctors no mind, Ms. Mann ordered food from local restaurants delivered beside. As she munched rebelliously, her blood sugars skyrocketed, requiring continuous insulin infusions. The staff could not track all the reckless carbohydrate ingestions. Her potassium towered with ongoing threats of cardiac arrest while the pulmonary fluid flooded air sacks, requiring daily dialysis.

Hospitalist Levi and nephrologist Chase insisted she adhere to a strict diabetic/renal diet monitored by the hospital dietician. They had a psychiatrist determine Ms. Mann fully capable of understanding the dire state of her condition and the repercussions of treatment noncompliance. Nursing supervisor Geoff intervened. Geoff declared that denying Ms. Mann the right to eat whatever she wanted in the hospital violated her personal rights. Levi and Chase persisted, giving Ms. Mann two options: comply with the recommendations so that she could be appropriately treated or leave.

Ms. Mann chose to leave.

■ ■ ■

Case 1:

Talk about defeating the purpose! Essentially, Mr. Mann's treatment was an academic exercise to deplete resources in a nonacademic facility.

Picture the field day medical attorneys would have if Mr. Mann deteriorated from respiratory failure on the very campus that welcomed his right to smoke while treating his unstable pulmonary state caused by smoking.

Case 2:

Nursing supervisor Geoff advocated for patients' rights to do whatever they please, wherever they please, however they please. So, according to Geoff's understanding of patients' rights, a patient does not need to comply with any of the rules set forth by any institution, even if that patient's desires contradict the institution's purpose to improve that patient's well-being. If Geoff had taken a second to consider the lethal ramifications, he may have realized that Ms. Mann had every right to exercise her personal rights outside of the hospital where the only harm and waste she would inflict would be upon herself. Instead, someone else in need of dialysis would have to wait until her chair was no longer occupied. Someone else in need of IV fluids or medication would have to wait until Ms. Mann's nurse finished addressing her self-induced complications. Should one person's rights be upheld at the expense of everyone else's, particularly when it serves whims of only that one?

Most importantly, Ms. Mann's rights opposed her contract to heal herself. Was not her acceptance of admission a contract to comply with the treatment plan and recommendations by medical providers?

Geoff was correct. Ms. Mann had her rights.

Levi and Chase were correct. Ms. Mann had her rights.

However, when defining rights, one must be certain the rights are campaigned within the right context: In medicine's treat-to-heal contract, Ms. Mann had one right – comply or leave.

brain dead – an epic failure

(A true story with a pinch of dramatization ... but only a pinch)

Some Hospital, Somewhere, Some World

The Executive Office:

"What?! What's with all the commotion?"

"We have a disaster on our hands!"

"What?! Fire? Crazed psychotic? What?! What's happening?"

"Something has happened in our system. Uh, um, there's a glitch *we* did to it! And, and, and..."

"What? Spit it out!"

"The EHR crashed!"

"Aw! Aw, Aw, $#1111111111111t!"

The Hospitalist Office:

Hospitalist Coordinator Clark stared blankly at the blank screen staring blankly at him. He urgently reshuffled the confused printouts he had shuffled thirty seconds before.

"Wha – What am I supposed to do with this? Those lists – These lists are useless! I don't know who's still here, who's been sent home, who came in overnight or where anyone is! These docs are going to kill me today! I can't create lists for them! They're just going to be headless chickens today! Damn!"

Clark frantically phoned the first of five unit clerks.

"I got to do what? ... Do you know how many rooms are in this place?"

"Gene, you are only responsible for your floor. The others will take care of theirs," Clark attempted.

"Do you know how many rooms are in this place? ... You really expect me to go room to room and tally who's left and who's still here? ... Seriously?! ... By myself? And what if they're off the floor? ... Seriously?! Do you know how long this will take me?"

"Hopefully not as long as your complaining. Please, Gene. I need to call the other floors now!"

Clark relived that exchange four more times with the remaining unit clerks. Hospitalist Site Leader Mitch swooned in on the tail end of Clark's final phone call.

"Mitch, I got the unit clerks tallying the patients on the floors, but I don't know anything about the admissions that came in after the crash. Could you find them?"

"Oh, okay. Uh, in the ER?"

"The ER, Radiology, the floors. They're just floating around here somewhere. Who knows? There's nothing on them. They could be anywhere."

"Yeah, okay. Yeah."

Mitch jostled off. The hospitalists began to trickle in.

Hospitalist Martin huffed at the news. With pinched lips he absorbed the impending doom awaiting on the floors. He brusquely accepted his piecemeal list from Clark and attacked the phones, calling every floor in search of his patients as well as any administrator he could plaster his petition on.

Hospitalist Skip, aptly named for his rounding prowess, sank slowly as he stared imploringly at the stoic computer screens. He never, ever during his entire career had to resort to manual noting. Sure, ages ago it had been the mainstay, but this is the new world. Who could do such a thing in this day and age? Where are the templates?! Skip mournfully draped his palm over a computer mouse then listlessly moved it about as he dejectedly trailed its aimless tracking across the screen. Worse still, this was Skip's first day of service. He knew no one, unlike Martin who was familiar with at least half his service. At most, thanks to periodic backup Business Continuity Access (BCA) computers, Skip had the last EHR snapshot of a few patients' information (like diagnoses, recent treatments, test results and vital signs). But, even with this abetting scrap, Skip had to stand in line and wait his turn. Only one BCA computer had been allotted per floor, and *everyone* needed it.

2 hours in:

Overhead Announcement:

"Doctors, nurses, case workers, emergency huddle for updates and reassessments, immediately!"

And now emergency huddling?! Skip was ready to bolt. Still he had an obligation; he had to bring home some bacon. So, off to the huddle he marched.

Secretly gleaming, hospitalist Oscar buzzed past frazzled supervisors, nurses, case managers, pharmacists, specialists and hospitalists. Returning to his corner after his huddle, as he facilely scribbled away, Oscar reveled in this serendipitous homage to the *good ol'e days* when documenting was much simpler. He basked in the freedom he once had many, many moons ago when he could compose his notes without electronic fettering. He too was starting his service that day, which, on a typical electronically bossed day, would take him well past the end of his shift to complete. Today, however, Oscar zipped from assessment to assessment dodging the bewildered others too preoccupied with bewilderment to hammer him with trivialities.

4 hours in:

Overhead Announcement:

"Doctors, nurses, case workers, emergency huddle for updates and reassessments, immediately!"

After that last huddle, unfortunately, Oscar was cornered by a bewildered. Hospitalist Milton followed the seemingly insouciant Oscar to his corner.

"Dude! What's up? Do you not see what's going on here? What's with you?" Milton demanded.

"Seeing patients just like you."

"But how? There's no EHR!"

"Yeah, but I can still write progress notes."

"Yeah, but how? You don't have any templates now. ... Or do you?" Milton pried rabidly.

"Uh, don't need one. See." Oscar showed Milton a note. "Just write it out."

"Can I borrow this. I want to make a copy. I haven't started my notes yet."

Meanwhile in the cardiology suite, cardiologist Pierce grew concerned that Ms. Mann's ongoing chest pain heralded an occluded cardiac artery. He contacted the catherization lab (Cath lab) for an emergency heart catherization (Cath) to open the artery and restore perfusion to the heart. Amid the hurried preparations, Pierce answered a summons to meet with Administration in the conference room. Administrator Klaus stared incredulously at Pierce.

"Why do you want to perform a procedure while the EHR is still down?"

"This woman needs this Cath if she is to live. She has left main disease that will shut *her* down if we don't Cath her as soon as possible. Don't worry. This is what I do, what I've done even before the EHR came about. There will be a detailed written report."

"What will you do if the patient has severe disease that needs surgical repair and must be transferred to a higher-level facility?"

"Just as it's always been done. We transfer the patient."

"Then how would you complete a discharge summary without an EHR?" Klaus finished smugly.

"I'd *write* one."

6 hours in:

> Overhead Announcement:
>
> > "Doctors, nurses, case workers, emergency huddle for updates and reassessments, immediately!"

Hospitalist Ryan shook his head in exasperation.

"Nope! Nope! Not doing it. Nope," Ryan grumbled into the air. "First they make this do-or-die call in the middle of my exam, then I had to rush through the patient, then I had to race to the conference room on the other side of the building, only to wait for Admin to figure out what they called us in there for. Then they wanna ask every single one of us what we are doing to deal with the crash and offer help they don't know how to give!" Ryan fumed to the captive silence. "Forty minutes lost to talking about working. No, no. I'm not doing it this time! How am I supposed to get patients what they need if I keep running off to meetings all the time? I've got to get my work done." The room empathized. Ryan gruffly sat down and sorted through his patient list, calling whomever he needed for information. Suddenly, he slammed the phone and slowly slid his hands from forehead to cheeks.

"YOU'VE GOT TO BE KIDDING ME!" he exclaimed.

Ryan could not discharge two medically stable patients, because their tests had been canceled, because *the EHR* said so.

In another, unsuspecting wing of the hospital ...

A Mr. Mann strolled into the laboratory department for his scheduled appointment. He was baffled when asked to fill out some paper form as opposed to the electronic registration to which he had been accustomed. The form was unfamiliar and long. Lab technician Zachary directed Mr. Mann to lie on the table for his procedure then left the room. Mr. Mann undressed, donned the immodest hospital gown, lay on the chilly table, and waited with a slight shiver.

Zachary perused the paper form detailing the procedure. After a few paragraphs, Zachary discovered it was the incorrect form. Usually, he never had to concern himself with forms: the computer took care of it. He asked lab assistant Trevor to get the correct form. Thirty minutes later, Trevor returned with shrugged shoulders and surrendered hands; he could not find the form. Lost, Zachary contacted Administrator Klaus. Klaus instructed Zachary to cancel Mr. Mann's procedure and all other nonemergent scheduled procedures until further notice.

Much, much, much later, Zachary returned to the shivering Mr. Mann with the update.

Smoldering, Mr. Mann slipped from his flimsy garb, hurtled it to the floor, yanked on his warm clothes, and stormed out.

8 hours in:

> Overhead Announcement:
>
>> *"Doctors, nurses, case workers, emergency huddle for updates and reassessments, immediately!"*

The hospitalists trudge through their respective duties. Skip, who usually skips through his day with an early departure, left work nearly three hours later than usual. With cramped fingers, fatigued limbs and demoralized spirits, Skip prayed the shutdown would not spill into another day. Oscar reviewed his checklist incredulously: he had finished EVERYTHING with two hours for thumb twiddling by the day's end.

Sometime in the wee hours of the night, over twenty-four hours later, the EHR came back to life.

...

The Aftermath:

The next morning, Skip shambled into the hospital. A sigh of gratitude twirled out of his chest as he stood among the familiar rap of clicking mice. Merrily rooting himself before a computer, Skip reviewed his patients' charts. Wait! One of his patients did not have the IV fluids and antibiotics he had ordered on paper yesterday! Those orders must have been overlooked, because they were not in the computer! Skip checked the nurses' notes. There was nothing there. No one thought it odd that a patient with a raging infection had no treatments. Petrified, Skip's gaze trailed slowly from the screen to the ceiling.

"If *she* didn't get her antibiotics, maybe Mr. Mann didn't get ..."

Overhead Announcement:

"*CODE 333!*

www.ingramcontent.com/pod-product-compliance
Lightning Source LLC
Chambersburg PA
CBHW051336200326
41519CB00026B/7449